THE
HEALTHY
SKIN
DIET

THIS BOOK IS DEDICATED TO
MY LOVING HUSBAND AND SON, MY FAMILY
AND THE MEMORY OF MY STRONG LITTLE MUM.

THE
HEALTHY
SKIN
DIET

RECIPES & 4-WEEK EATING PLAN TO SUPPORT SKIN HEALTH & HEALING AT ANY AGE

Geraldine Georgeou

murdoch books

Sydney | London

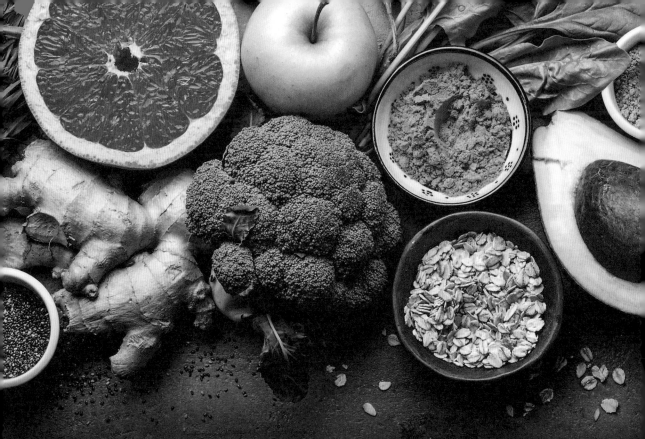

CONTENTS

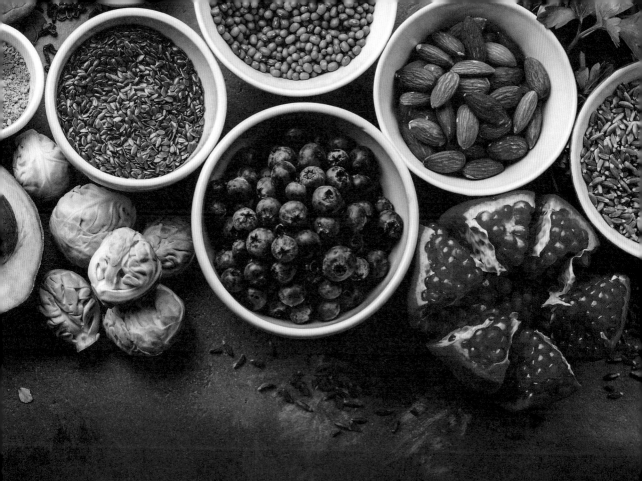

INTRODUCTION:
About Geraldine

If you're a dietitian, and your livelihood is based around helping others achieve their health goals, it's hard to admit when you're not in control of your own body.

For years I struggled with polycystic ovarian syndrome (PCOS), its secondary effect of fluctuating weight, and the confusion and guilt that comes with feeling that I 'should know better'. The uphill battle against my own hormones had an impact on my skin and hair, as well as on my confidence when working with patients. So, for me, this isn't just a book: it has been a lifelong journey towards discovering the true power behind nutrition.

Over the years I've had the privilege of working alongside world leaders in the medical fields of endocrinology, dermatology and gastroenterology. As exciting new science continues to emerge, we have realised the true impact of insulin resistance, inflammation, PCOS, gluten intolerance, coeliac disease and the ways in which food chemicals affect the skin. Today, together with knowing a patient's health situation and addressing both nutrition and any underlying medical conditions, we can improve not only their skin, but also their overall health.

'Look good, feel good' is my mantra. My own experience, while I was also providing dietetic advice to others over the years, has helped me give simple, practical eating and nutrition advice for individuals with problem skin; advice that can be embraced by the entire family. I hope to help take the heartache out of what can be, for many, an upsetting and life-limiting problem.

The cliché 'you are what you eat' is absolutely true. I see it every day in practice, and yet somehow it's never been explored from the perspective of skin. As the largest organ in the body, skin can benefit from the same nutrition we get from foods that have a positive effect on our heart and other major organs, and even on diabetes.

This book is not a diagnostic tool and should not be used as a substitute for individual medical advice. Rather, it can be used as a general guide to help readers understand possible connections between their skin and their diet, which should be tailored to suit their individual medical and nutritional needs.

From macronutrients and 'balanced eating', to micronutrients and functional nutrients, I will show you how easy it is to make better food choices and nutritional changes that will support glowing skin and overall better health. My aim is to offer you scientific research on a plate for breakfast, lunch and dinner. I want to give you practical ways to help protect your skin from free radicals caused by sun exposure, by increasing your intake of antioxidants such as vitamins C and E. And I'd like to show you how to improve the integrity of your skin, hair and nails by harnessing the natural potential of B vitamins, biotin and vitamin A. I will also discuss how to use pre- and probiotics alongside other anti-inflammatory nutrients to effectively combat conditions such as eczema, rashes, acne and psoriasis.

I hope you, and your whole family, will come back to this book time and time again, and discover new things as you move through your health journey to better, glowing skin.

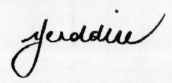

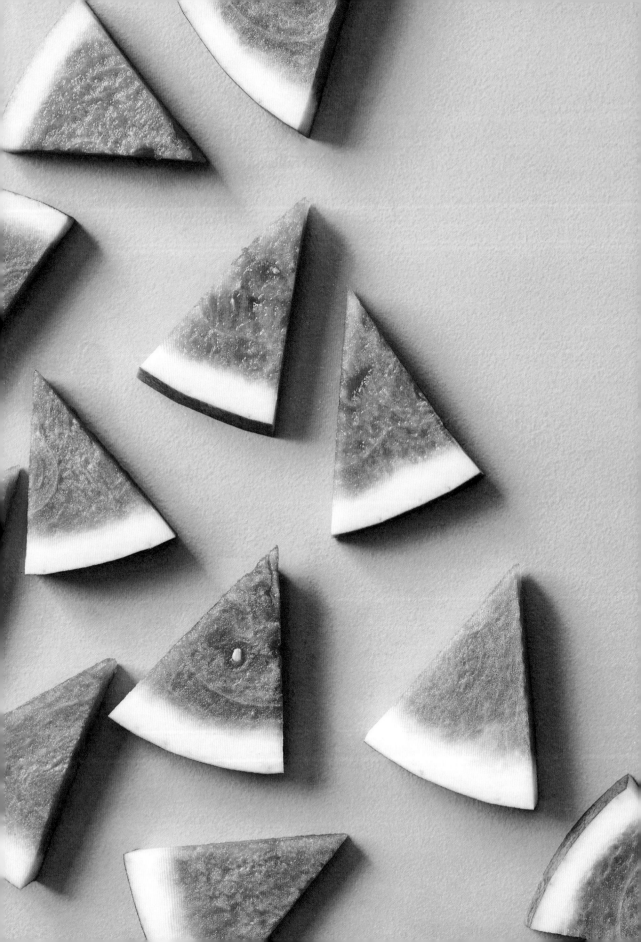

CHAPTER 1

ALL ABOUT SKIN

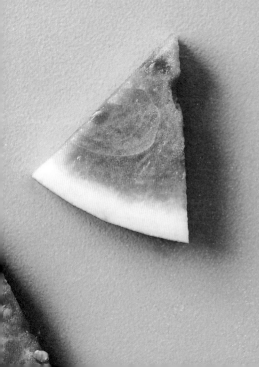

THE SKIN SYSTEM

Skin is an organ — the largest organ of the body — comprising around 15 per cent of your bodyweight. In textbooks you will see it referred to as the 'integumentary system', derived from the Latin word *integumentum*, which means 'covering'.

Just as you have a cardiovascular system and a gastrointestinal system, the skin is a system of its own. The skin system includes hair follicles and hair, nails, sebaceous (oil) glands and sweat glands, so, as you can imagine, if you've got one problem with your skin, such as on your face, it could be connected with another part of your integumentary system. It makes sense that we need to understand how skin works with all the other organs and systems in the body; how it can influence your moods and self-confidence; and why worrying about what you put *on* your skin is only half the answer to helping it stay healthy.

Just as the eyes are said to be the window to the soul, I consider your skin to be the window to your health, yet we often ignore what the body is trying to tell us. We breezily dismiss its messages as 'just a rash', 'a bit of eczema' or 'another annoying breakout', and ignore or minimise what these symptoms might really be indicating. In fact, changes in your skin can often be the first hint of an underlying health issue.

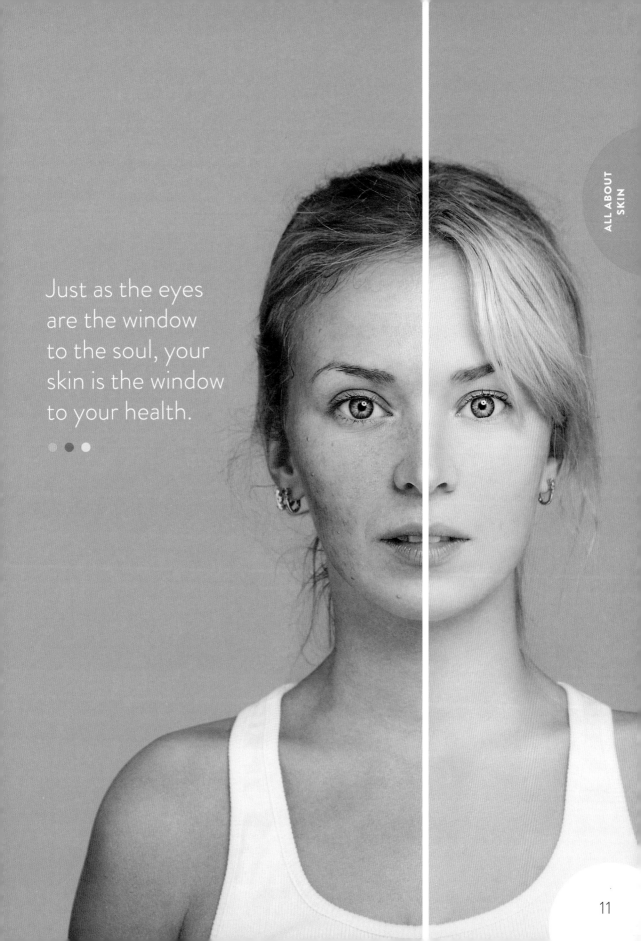

Just as the eyes
are the window
to the soul, your
skin is the window
to your health.

Layers of the skin

Let's think of the skin as a cake with several layers that have many functions and roles to play. It is made up of three main layers: the 'epidermis', 'dermis' and 'subcutaneous' layers. The **epidermis** is a thin, outer, waterproof barrier that keeps your insides in and the outside world out. It is the visible part of the skin and it's the layer that makes melanin, which is what gives skin its pigment. It's thinner in some areas, such as your eyelids, and much thicker on the soles of your feet, allowing parts of the body to have different functions and levels of protection. The epidermis is where your hair follicles, sweat glands and sebaceous (oil) glands open onto the surface.

OXIDATIVE STRESS

You might have heard of free radicals? These unstable molecules can damage cells, leading to ageing and diseases such as cancer. They occur when we're exposed to pollutants such as smoking, ozone, and UV rays from the sun. The antioxidant system is in charge of managing free radicals; however, if the system becomes unbalanced with too many free radicals, this is known as oxidative stress.

The **dermis** layer lies underneath the epidermis and it provides the 'architecture of youth'. It is a much thicker layer and carries out many functions. The dermis houses the base of the sweat glands, hair follicles, sebaceous glands and it contains nerve endings, too. It uses specialised proteins called collagen and elastin to give your skin the plump, dewy freshness that everyone over the age of 30 seems to be forever chasing!

You have around three million sweat glands in your skin, which help regulate body temperature. Sebaceous glands secrete an oil called sebum to lubricate skin, keeping it soft and supple; sebum also has antifungal and antibacterial properties to help prevent infections. Sebum has a bad reputation as being responsible for the pimples that can pop up at inconvenient times during your life cycle (whether you're young or old).

The dermis is about much more than how you look: the nerve endings it contains provide sensory feedback to your brain,

● ● ●

Think of the skin as a cake with three different layers.

and they interpret temperature, pressure, touch, vibration, pain and itching. And when you are exposed to the sun's ultra-violet radiation, the dermis synthesises its own vitamin D, which enables your body to absorb calcium and phosphorus.

Below the dermis you'll find the third layer, **subcutaneous fat**, which is made up of collagen fibres and fat cells. This layer of fat protects your organs from injury or trauma, chemicals, bacteria, parasites and infection, and especially assists with insulation and regulating your body temperature. A fat layer might not sound too sexy, but when it comes to skin it is incredibly important. I've seen many patients with damaged subcutaneous skin from extreme dieting and yo-yo weight loss: if this layer of fat shrinks and loses its plumpness, it can age you dramatically.

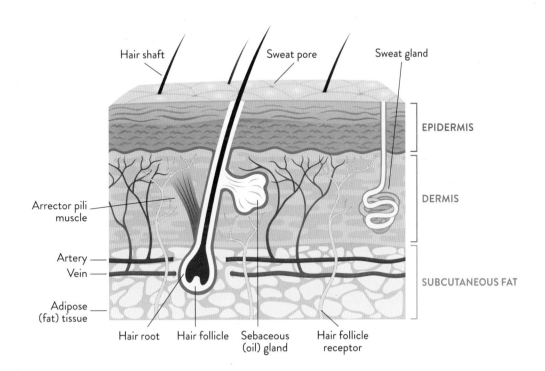

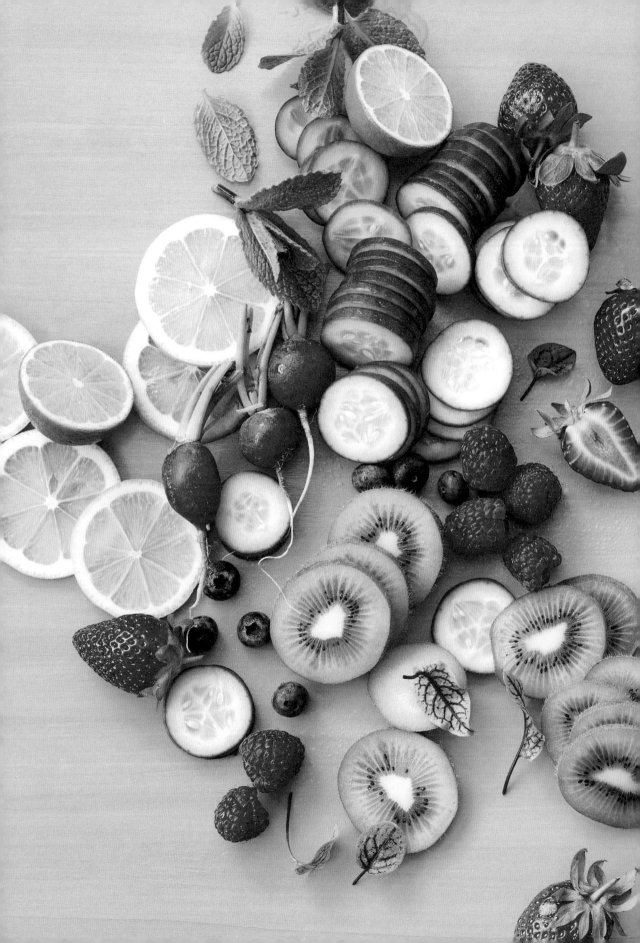

Skin changes from the sun

While the most obvious effect of sun damage is its effects on skin ageing — such as wrinkles and sun spots — the sun can have more sinister effects. Too much exposure to the sun's UV rays can damage skin cells, causing skin cancer to occur. Australia, where I live, has one of the highest rates of skin cancer in the world: around 12,000 people are diagnosed and 2000 people die every year from this almost entirely preventable disease.

UV LIGHT When you're exposed to UV light your skin produces melanin, the dark pigment in the epidermis layer. The extra melanin darkens your skin, creating a suntan — this is your body's attempt to block the sun's UV rays. Most people can't produce enough melanin to protect their skin from exposure and their skin turns red, swells and 'burns'. Repeated burning can lead to premature ageing — from wrinkles, discoloured skin spots, rough skin — and skin cancer.

THREE TYPES OF SKIN CANCER There are three main types of skin cancer: basal cell carcinoma, squamous cell carcinoma and, the most dangerous, melanoma. If you have concerns about any suspicious spots on your skin, visit your GP who can assess the level of risk and also give advice on early detection and treatment.

CHECK YOUR SKIN Get to know your skin and what is normal for you, so that you notice any changes. Skin cancers often don't display any symptoms, such as pain or itching, and are usually seen, rather than felt. Develop a regular habit of checking your skin for new spots and changes to existing freckles or moles. The good news is that being sun smart can be a simple and effective way to reduce the risk of developing any type of skin cancer. For more information on how to protect your skin from the sun, go to your country's national cancer website and search for 'preventing skin cancer'.

Skin changes over your lifetime

Fight it as we try, skin changes and ages just as consistently as we do. Babies remain blissfully unaware of their smooth-as-butter bottoms and enviable complexions, only to inevitably grow into angsty acne-prone teenagers. Eventually we develop those fine lines that are signs of our mortality, and wrinkles and sun damage tell the story of how we have lived our lives. But what is happening beneath the surface that causes skin to change in appearance?

Everything is a race against the clock. Both internal and external factors are responsible for the changes that occur over a lifetime. Internally, genetics determine the speed at which your skin ages. Over time, cell turnover slows down and sebum production and collagen production decline, leading to thinning, drying skin and uneven pigmentation. Since collagen makes up around 70 per cent of the dermis,

and is what gives your skin its supple youthful appearance, it's important you look after it, both inside and out. As you age and your collagen production slows, the subcutaneous fat (lipid) layer of your skin reduces and your skin's water-holding ability diminishes. This explains why skin loses volume and plumpness as you age, becoming rougher and less elastic. At a functional level, your skin becomes less effective at healing wounds, and at acting as a protective barrier, as you age.

On top of this, excessive sun exposure and the effects of gravity on the ageing face lead to wrinkles (often kindly referred to as 'smile lines'). And there are lifestyle factors, such as tobacco smoking, which is toxic to cells, and unprotected exposure to the sun or the use of tanning beds, which serve to accelerate the ageing process and place you at risk of skin cancer.

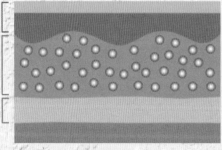

EPIDERMIS

YOUTHFUL DERMIS WITH COLLAGEN

FAT (LIPID) LAYER

YOUTHFUL SKIN

AGEING SKIN

Less supportive collagen in the ageing dermis means the epidermis above collapses and folds, forming wrinkles.

Hormones & skin

We can't talk about skin without talking about hormones ... the body's invisible messengers that can create harmony or havoc at every stage of life. The embarrassing patch of hair in an odd place, the irrational mood swings, pimples and even boils, up-and-down hunger, hot flushes ... all hormones. But how?

Hormones are the chemical messengers of our body. They are produced by specialist cells, often in the endocrine glands, and travel through the bloodstream, controlling all the systems of the body. They signal and communicate to help the body regulate its many different functions, such as digestion, sex and reproduction, sleeping, relaxing, concentrating, respiration, growth, movement, managing stress, excretion, lactation and many, many more.

MENOPAUSE & SKIN A woman's skin changes again when she goes through a hormonal transition later in life: menopause. During menopause, skin thickness decreases. Menopause contributes to a decrease in the three ingredients that keep skin looking young and healthy: collagen production slows and the replenishment rate of elastin cells and hyaluronic acid declines. Furthermore, oestrogen levels drop markedly during menopause, to the detriment of your skin's capacity to hold water and remain plump and full. These factors, in addition to those mentioned earlier — such as sun exposure, gravity, tobacco use and the genetic speed at which each individual's skin ages — cause thinner, sagging skin, lines and wrinkles. It is important to keep well nourished if you want to lessen the impact of ageing, and food for your skin will be explored later in detail.

Insulin & insulin resistance

One of the body's most important and well-examined hormones is insulin; I'll mention it a lot. Insulin is the hormone that allows the cells of your body to transport and use sugar (glucose) from the carbohydrates you've eaten. Your body's cells need this sugar to give them energy, but sugar can't enter the cells directly: insulin is the chemical messenger that signals to cells to absorb sugar from the bloodstream. It is often described as a 'key' that is used to unlock cells and let in the sugar. In this way insulin keeps the amount of sugar in your bloodstream at the right level. When you eat, and the level of sugar in your blood rises, the cells in your pancreas release more insulin into your blood. Foods that contain unrefined sugars thus trigger your pancreas to release lots of insulin.

If you have eaten more sugar than your body needs, insulin helps store it in the liver to be released when your supplies are low (perhaps when you're exercising). If your body doesn't produce enough insulin, or your cells become resistant to it, you can develop high blood sugar.

Type 1 diabetics can't make insulin, because the cells in their pancreas are faulty and they need insulin injections to help their body process glucose. Type 2 diabetics have become resistant to insulin. They might be able to manage this with

A LIFETIME OF INSULIN

Insulin affects us all our lives, changing its role and efficiency at different times. Insulin problems, such as insulin resistance, are often seen as just 'normal changes' in the body and not picked up. Parts of this timeline might feel familiar for readers.

PUBERTY
You grow quicker than your peers, maybe become a little chubby around this time, plus have oily hair and skin. Females might start their periods earlier than their peers.

OLDER TEENAGER
Males might battle midriff weight, increased breast tissue (man boobs), acne and oily hair. Females might have irregular or painful periods or not get them at all, and then be put on the pill to regulate them. When you come off the pill you battle acne, excess body hair and weight but blame 'partying' and lifestyle.

changes to diet and exercise, or could need medicine or insulin injections to help control their blood sugar levels.

If you become insulin resistant, it means that your body produces insulin but your cells can no longer recognise it, which can leave the sugar in your bloodstream, rather than getting it into your muscles and other body parts. So then your body keeps making more insulin. At this stage you might need medication to help your insulin transport sugar better, or you might be able to adjust what you eat to stop your body triggering more insulin than you need. An endocrine test can confirm your underlying insulin levels.

In the following chapters you will see that there is a common theme between your skin, your hormones and your insulin function over your lifetime. The fact that you are what you eat might be only half the story. How you eat, and how your hormones respond — causing insulin resistance — might help explain a variety of skin conditions. Research has found links between diet and 'teenage' acne, polycystic ovarian syndrome (PCOS), acne rosacea, menopause, pigmentation, psoriasis, eczema, hirsutism (excess body hair), dermatitis, alopecia and even random skin tags. I will explore these in greater detail in Chapter 4.

TWENTIES & BEYOND

You get married or settle down. You lose weight for the celebration, but it creeps back on, plus more. You develop rashes — psoriasis, eczema or ongoing acne. Males get a beer belly and male-pattern hair loss. Females might have trouble getting pregnant or be diagnosed with PCOS, or fall pregnant and develop gestational diabetes and acne.

MIDLIFE

As you age, lean body mass changes, with loss of muscle and increased body fat, plus annoying skin tags. You might have a family history of diabetes, stroke, gout, fatty liver, arthritis and heart disease. Your midriff weight might increase and women develop a form of adult acne — rosacea — at menopause.

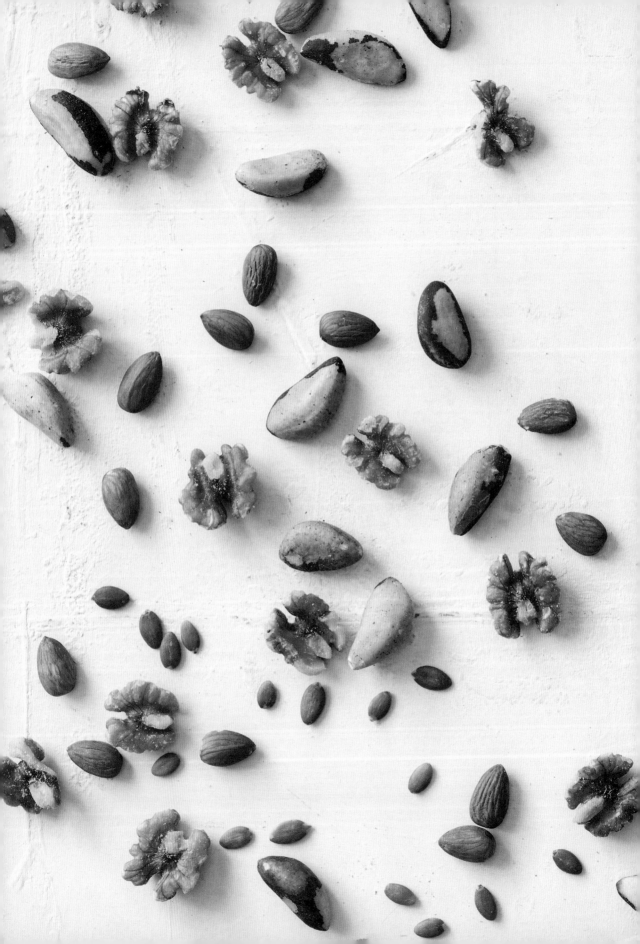

CHAPTER 2

NUTRITION: YOUR SKIN'S SECRET WEAPON

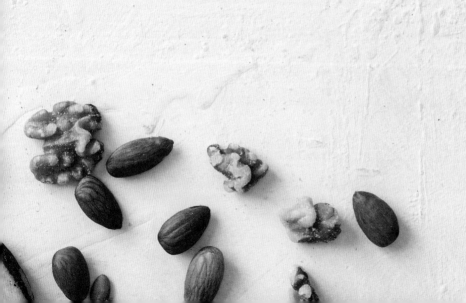

FEEDING YOUR SKIN

All foods are made up of a combination of macronutrients and micronutrients. As food passes through our body — from mouth, to stomach, to gut — it is used for fuel or for nutrition. Macronutrients are broken down to use as energy and fuel, the building blocks of our cells and essential fatty acids. Micronutrients, such as vitamins and minerals, are the functional nutrients used to keep cells healthy. Nutrition plays a huge role in managing skin and skin health.

Carbohydrates

Carbohydrates are the body's first source of fuel; cutting out carbs can make you feel lethargic, irritable and weak, and even crave sugar. A lot of people these days seem to view carbs as 'the enemy'. Many people ask me, 'Can I just cut out carbohydrates or grains?' I consider this impossible to sustain over a long period of time: you will lack energy and you will not meet your daily fibre requirement. It is also quite hard to make a family meal without an entire food group: there would be no more sandwiches, no more roast dinners with pumpkin and potatoes ... How will you fill up a growing teenage son?

Carbs can be part of a healthy meal plan, but portion size is the key: look at the meal plans for guidance here, but remember that everyone has different nutritional needs, depending on their age and energy requirements. Wholegrain breads, wholegrain cereals, pasta, basmati rice and starchy vegetables such as potatoes, sweet potatoes, peas and corn can be included in your meals and snacks. In addition to these foods, fruits, legumes, reduced-fat milk and reduced-fat yoghurt are also good sources of carbohydrate that can be included in meals.

We all know that sugar and refined carbohydrates are very dense and rich in 'fuel' and, if overconsumed, can lead to weight gain, a rise in blood sugar levels and a fluctuation of the hormones related to acne, psoriasis and inflammation.

But using the words sugar and carbohydrates in the same sentence does not mean they have the same effect on the body. The truth is, not all carbohydrates are equal; it depends completely on the meal and the portion. Carbohydrates can also be ranked by their rate of absorption into the bloodstream; this is known as their glycaemic index (GI).

The glycaemic index is a ranking of carbohydrates, based on their immediate effect on blood sugar levels graded from 0–100 after consumption. It compares the carbohydrate value of foods, gram for gram. Carbohydrates that break down quickly during digestion, releasing glucose quickly into the bloodstream, have the highest GI. Carbohydrates that break down slowly, releasing glucose gradually into the bloodstream, have a lower GI.

The benefit of low-GI foods is that the slow release of glucose into the bloodstream helps keep you feeling fuller for longer and provides longer-lasting energy (particularly when combined with lean protein and good fats, plus vegetables). Sugar (or, more precisely, glucose) is a high-GI carbohydrate; it is digested quickly and can provide your body with energy immediately. This is sometimes useful (our ancient ancestors needed fast energy to fuel their fight-or-flight response when danger was near); however, the quick release of sugar into the bloodstream can also trigger a cascade of physiological and hormonal events that might ultimately cause inflammation.

The idea that diet 'feeds our skin' might have once been dismissed as a fairytale, but over the past decade there has been increasing evidence that what we eat — and, more specifically, the sugar that we consume — really does show up on our skin. The intake of sugar, and other high-GI carbohydrate foods, has been shown to increase the levels of insulin in the bloodstream, which can trigger hormonal disturbances such as an increase of testosterone production. The rise in male hormone can then lead to an increase in the production of oil from glands in your skin and drive inflammatory processes.

An eating plan that includes less sugar, more low-GI carbohydrates, balanced protein and controlled fat appears to have a positive effect on skin. A 2007 Australian study, *Acne in Adolescence,* showed that young men who followed a low-GI diet experienced significant healing of acne.

It's important to note that a high sugar intake can also disrupt the gut microbiome, leading to gastrointestinal inflammation, which also links to a higher incidence of skin issues.

Refined, highly processed carbohydrates, especially those put into a package that is palatable and encourages overconsumption — for example, crisps, lollies and chocolate — can be considered to be 'bad carbo-hydrates'. Carbohydrates in their natural state (as found in nature) are not refined. It is important to remember that many populations around the world maintain good health on higher carbohydrate diets of natural and unprocessed foods, such as rice.

CUTTING CARBS

Cutting out healthy carbs, such as wholegrain bread and cereals, can be dangerous to your body. They provide:

> your primary source of energy, especially for your brain

> nutrients your body needs, such as vitamin C, folate and B group vitamins

> a great source of fibre – good carb sources of fibre include legumes, wholegrain breads and cereals, fruits and vegetables

> an important aid to digestion — they are a source of fuel for your gastrointestinal microbiome

Protein

Protein is the building block of muscles, skin, keratin in hair, nails, enzymes and hormones, and it plays an essential role in all body tissues. It is the second most common compound in the body, after water. It is used for growth and repair of cells and tissues in the body, so it is important to include protein in every meal to allow for these processes. It's important too that a healthy balance of protein and carbohydrates are included in your diet.

Protein foods play a major role in assisting us to feel full after a meal. With a similar energy content per gram to carbohydrates, protein requires more time to break down, because of its molecular composition. Protein is made up of long chains of peptides, formed by lots of building blocks called amino acids; these need to be broken down before they can enter the bloodstream and be used by the body. 'Complete proteins' contain nine essential amino acids.

When we talk about proteins, we often mean meats such as chicken, fish, beef, lamb and pork, as well as meat alternatives such as nuts and eggs. We can't forget about those plant foods that are also good sources of protein, such as tofu, beans, lentils and other legumes. Only three of these plant sources — buckwheat, quinoa and soy — are 'complete proteins'. Dairy products — including milk, cheese and yoghurt — are also rich sources of protein. Other plant-based sources such as nuts and seeds are incomplete proteins, so if you eat only plant-based foods you need to choose a variety to make sure your body's needs are met.

It is important with any food group to encompass a wide variety of sources in your diet. We need to aim for between two and three serves of meat and meat alternatives per week (this will be dependent on your age, gender and activity level and each country has government guidelines). Lean cuts of meat are recommended to ensure that you aren't eating too much saturated fat, which would raise your bad cholesterol levels. (This is the reason why 'lite' and reduced-fat dairy products are recommended for adults.) Removing the skin from chicken and trimming the fat from red meat before cooking will also reduce the amount of saturated fat you eat, of course.

By including a balance of lean protein with unrefined carbohydrates and good fats, such as grilled chicken breast combined with a baked sweet potato and leafy salad with avocado and tomato, we are able to control the release of sugars into the bloodstream after digestion, therefore controlling insulin production. As we've seen, if there is an elevated level of insulin circulating in the body, this can promote inflammation and exacerbate the hormones associated with skin problems. Hence, protein is vitally important to weight control and skin health.

Fats

These days fats are seen as an essential food in our daily diet. Incorporating healthy fats in what you eat will provide vitamins A, D, E and K, which are essential nutrients for general health and wellbeing and are also important for promoting healthy skin.

Adding good fats such as mono- and polyunsaturated fats (olive oil, avocado oil, rice bran oil, nut oils) to your diet helps cardiac health and good cholesterol production. It also helps to promote a low glycaemic response, which delays the time your body takes to break down food and increases satiety and the feeling of fullness. All of which means that you are less likely to get the munchies and crave sugar.

A study called *Skin Wrinkling: Can Food Make a Difference?*, published in February 2001, found 'that subjects with a higher intake of vegetables, olive oil, and monounsaturated fat and legumes, but a lower intake of milk/dairy products, butter, margarine and sugar products had less skin wrinkling in a sun-exposed site'. It was suggested that this might be due to lower oxidative stress with a healthy diet — the body isn't inflamed by the chemical challenges of trying to process unhealthy foods, so cutting them out reduces the cell damage from within.

Saturated fats from meat and dairy can increase your risk of heart disease and bowel cancer. Trans fatty acids, which are fats produced from industrial processed foods, are often found in commercial fried foods, cakes, pastries and some crackers. They have been shown in studies to be harmful to skin health, promoting oxidative damage when exposed to UV radiation.

Good sources of added fats include extra virgin olive oil on your salads, or even avocado oil. Avocado and nuts are great sources of monounsaturated fats that can easily be included in your daily intake; they can really add flavour and texture and satiety to your meals. Don't forget there are other types of fats, such as rice bran oil, which we know has a very high smoking point (the temperature to which it can be heated), which means it won't denature or break down when you're cooking and will maintain its healthy fat status.

Micronutrients

It is important to understand how functional micronutrients affect your skin, but this doesn't make supplements, pills and potions your gateway to the perfect complexion. Your secret weapon is in the recipe section of this book, which has been formulated to incorporate into your diet all the micronutrients that promote healthy and radiant skin.

VITAMIN A:
A IS FOR ANTIOXIDANT

Vitamin A is a fat-soluble vitamin, important for producing healthy skin cells.

It is an antioxidant that supports the production of collagen and elastin fibres, and helps protect against redness and pigmentation from sun damage. Not getting enough vitamin A can lead to dry skin and slower healing of wounds. Betacarotene is the red–orange pigment, found in plenty of fruit and vegetables, which then converts to vitamin A in the body. Some excellent sources of beta-carotene are sweet potatoes, carrots, pumpkin and dark leafy greens such as kale and spinach.

VITAMIN B7:
HEALTHY SKIN COENZYME

Biotin, also known as B7, is one of the eight B vitamins that help us metabolise food for energy. Biotin is water soluble, so can't be stored in the body; instead, it has to be consumed every day. It's important for skin, hair and nail health and, although it is fairly uncommon to have a biotin deficiency, not getting enough vitamin B7 is associated with brittle nails, hair loss, and red, itchy, scaly rashes on the scalp. Biotin is found in abundance in many different foods, including yeast, brown rice, organ meats (liver and kidney), eggs and nuts.

CALCIUM:
THERE'S A GLASS AND A HALF IN EVERY ONE OF US!

Calcium is not only vital for strong, healthy bones, it also helps the outermost layer of our skin to grow and repair, by regulating the production of sebum to hydrate and maintain moisture in the skin. In addition to milk and yoghurt, you can also get calcium from chia seeds, almonds, tinned sardines and salmon (with bones), beans and lentils.

VITAMIN C:
FROM THE INSIDE OUT

It is quite well known that vitamin C plays a crucial role in collagen synthesis and protection against sun damage from UV rays. In recent times, topical skin treatments with vitamin C have become very popular; however, in my opinion, it is better to focus on getting adequate nutritional vitamin C so it can work its magic from within. Ingredients rich in vitamin C include capsicum (pepper), broccoli, tomato, parsley, guava, acerola (Barbados cherry) and blackcurrants.

COPPER:
CRAFTING COLLAGEN

Copper is another antioxidant that protects skin from sun damage. This mineral is known to stimulate collagen maturation, therefore maintaining the skin's thickness and elasticity. Copper helps control melanin synthesis, which gives our skin and hair their natural pigments. A severe copper deficiency can cause premature greyness. To get a good hit of copper, include liver, nuts, seeds, dark leafy greens, dark chocolate and chickpeas in your diet.

VITAMIN D:
THE WARRIOR FOOD

An adequate vitamin D level is important for wound healing and for soothing inflammation, but it's also an important player in healthy immunity. We all now know the importance of limiting time in the sun to avoid damage to our skin from harmful UV rays; however, we do need regular small doses of sunshine because sun exposure is also our primary source of vitamin D. Although we get most of our vitamin D from sun exposure, we can also obtain small amounts from foods such as mushrooms, tuna, salmon, egg yolks and liver.

VITAMIN E:
YOUR NATURAL SKIN BOOSTER

Our skin delivers vitamin E from the blood to the surface through sebum, which it uses as a sort of transport mechanism. Those people with oily skin — or even just one part of the body, such as the face, that produces more oil — have higher concentrations of vitamin E in their dermis and epidermis. Vitamin E's anti-inflammatory and antioxidant properties support immune function and skin health, and protect against UV damage; however, hormonal teenage overproduction of sebum can also lead to clogged pores and acne, so you may need to regulate your insulin levels to help with hormone production. Foods that are naturally high in vitamin E are sunflower seeds, avocado and nuts, such as almonds and peanuts.

IRON:
BODY ARMOUR AGAINST STRESS

In terms of skin health, iron is important for wound healing, combating oxidative stress and preventing damage from UV rays. When we don't have enough iron, our skin can appear paler and bruise more easily, nails might be brittle and dry, and hair may lack shine or even begin to fall out. The best and most efficient dietary sources of iron are animal products, namely red meat (which gives us haem iron); however, plant foods such as spinach, broccoli, lentils, beans, dried fruit, nuts and seeds are good sources of non-haem iron. Non-haem iron is harder for our bodies to digest because the fibre in the food prohibits its absorption. Thus we need to consume a far greater volume of the food to get the same nutrition; for example, two cups of boiled spinach contain the same amount of iron as 100g of lean red meat. We can improve iron absorption, especially of non-haem iron, by eating these foods with vitamin C–rich foods. It's also important to note that some foods, such as coffee, tea, wine and calcium-rich foods, can reduce iron absorption. So, if increasing iron is your goal, be sure to drink those separately, rather than at mealtimes.

OMEGA-3:
NOT JUST FOR BRAIN HEALTH

Omega-3 fatty acids — including DHA and EPA — are inflammation busters, keeping the skin hydrated by controlling oil production, fighting early signs of ageing and, again, protecting skin from sun damage. Oily fish is your best source, including salmon, tuna and swordfish; however, foods such as chia seeds, walnuts and flaxseeds are also great dietary sources of omega-3.

SELENIUM:
A POWERFUL MINERAL

Although we don't need much selenium, this essential mineral helps skin to fight against infection, reduces inflammation and prevents oxidative stress from sun exposure. Get selenium into your diet with seafood, brown rice and brazil nuts — just a single brazil nut contains more than the recommended daily intake.

SILICA:
THE MASTER BUILDER

Silica — the building block of skin, hair and nails — is important for wound healing and keeping the skin firm by helping with collagen production. Not having enough silica can lead to weak nails and dull, brittle hair, which is why it's used in so many herbal 'skin, hair and nail' formulations. Silica-rich foods include leeks, green beans, strawberries, cucumbers, celery, mango and asparagus.

ZINC:
MORE THAN JUST SUN PROTECTION

Zinc is one of the most touted skin-health minerals and for good reason: it is anti-inflammatory, protects from sun damage and exhibits antimicrobial action. There is some evidence that taking zinc supplements can help with acne (likely due to its wound healing and anti-microbial properties). Zinc is present in many foods, such as oysters, legumes, seeds, nuts, eggs and wholegrains.

Other buzz nutrients

COLLAGEN: **BONE BROTH**

Collagen is a protein found abundantly in the body: it is the main building block for skin. Collagen has received a lot of attention in recent decades, as it underpins a youthful, plump skin appearance and is essential for skin repair. Unfortunately, collagen — often found in bone broth — is not a complete protein. This means that when it's ingested as part of the diet it gets broken down and therefore doesn't reach the skin as actual collagen.

One research study has shown that the ingestion of proline (a component of collagen) might improve the elasticity of aged skin, but does not affect the skin's antioxidant capacity. This small study suggested that collagen peptides from bovine bone and proline could become a dietary supplement against skin ageing.

Further research about bioactive collagen peptides taken as supplements has shown them to stimulate the body's own collagen metabolism. Positive skin benefits include improved skin structure, reduced cellulite due to the improvement in the integrity of the dermis layer, and even improved nail growth.

I recommend a balanced diet with good sources of protein such as salmon, eggs, lean meats, lentils, nuts, seeds and seafood to help improve skin health and integrity. This will not only supply nutrients to the dermis (the thick layer of living tissue in the skin that lies below the epidermis), but promote naturally produced collagen as well.

CHLORELLA: **EATING GREEN**

This common single-celled green alga is what is found in stagnant water, turning it green. There are many species of *Chlorella*; and, despite the 'yuck' factor, it is enriched with nutrients, vitamins, minerals and chlorophyll and is often used as traditional medicine in the management of some inflammation-related diseases.

There are small studies of oral intake and topical administrations of *Chlorella* in mice, which showed improvement of skin inflammation and healing, and beneficial effects on skin lesions. More research into the role of these algae is needed, with human clinical studies required to confirm if it is truly a safe and effective treatment for skin.

CURCUMIN: **NATURE'S GOLD**

The active component in turmeric, curcumin has made a name for itself as a potent antioxidant and anti-inflammatory. Although evidence is not yet rock solid, we have a pretty good understanding that curcumin is beneficial in treating a number of diseases. It has shown promise as a psoriasis treatment, and is effective as a topical gel for reducing dryness, redness and plaque thickness. As an oral formulation, curcumin is effective compared to placebo and some people have improved their psoriasis by using it.

Other research suggests curcumin can reduce the time taken for wounds to heal, improve collagen production and increase the density of collagen-producing cells in wounds, making it useful for healing.

SPIRULINA: **GREENISH & BLUE**

Arthrospira (formerly *Spirulina*) *platensis* (AP) is a blue–green algae that contains approximately 70 per cent protein. It is also a source of B vitamins, especially B12 and pro-vitamin A (betacarotene), and minerals, especially iron. Rich in phenolic acids, tocopherols, carotene, ascorbic acid and gamma linolenic acid (GLA), spirulina is highly bioavailable, as the plant cell walls are easily digested.

It has sparked quite a lot of interest as a possible food supplement to nourish the skin. AP has been shown, in several small studies, to have antioxidant properties, to give protection from viruses and to inhibit the growth of multi-resistant bacteria. It has displayed possible anti-cancer activity in oral cancer, melanoma and in UV-induced non-melanoma skin cancer; however, more research is needed.

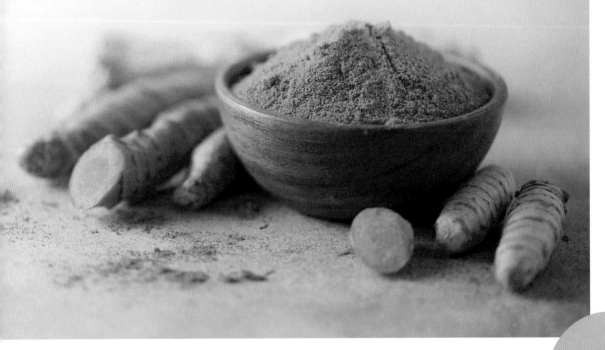

Food allergies & intolerances

Today, when a rash pops up out of nowhere, your first thought might be: 'What have I eaten?' Especially for parents: gone are the days when there was one kid in the school who was allergic to peanuts; now it's tricky to bring a birthday cake into class unless it's wheat-, lactose-, egg- and nut-free. The great debate of 'should' or 'shouldn't' perpetually fuels media controversy over allergies, saturates social media and polarises dinner tables. It's no wonder we don't trust ourselves to know how to eat anymore. Which begs the question: has the number of people with food allergies actually increased? Or is it a phenomenon of self-conscious dietary restriction?

Where I live, in Australia, we have one of the highest rates of food allergies in the world, with a 41 per cent increase in the risk of anaphylaxis reported between 2009 and 2014. In my own practice in Sydney I have seen more children presenting with insatiably itchy, red, scaly rashes, which often trigger guilt and self-doubt in the parents. The cause of the increase is uncertain, but research is beginning to explain how food allergies might have a role to play in eczema and atopic dermatitis. This is not to suggest that everyone with skin problems should eliminate peanuts, cow's milk and eggs, but it might be something you could investigate with the help of a dietitian.

There is, however, no dirtier word than 'gluten' in the public arena right now. To the shock of every baby boomer out there who was raised entirely on sandwiches, more and more people are jumping on the cauliflower-pizza-base bandwagon. But is there any evidence to suggest that anyone *without coeliac disease* should ditch gluten for their health? The overarching answer is no. Going gluten free without a diagnosis and expert help may provide no benefit. In fact, it can actually result in nutritional deficiencies and lower-fibre diets.

However, there *is* research to support the claim that a cohort of people have 'non-coeliac gluten sensitivity'. These people are intolerant to gluten and experience many of the symptoms that a sufferer of coeliac disease might get from ingesting gluten: diarrhoea, bloating, abdominal pain, fatigue and brain fog. They don't, however, experience permanent intestinal damage from eating gluten, like those with

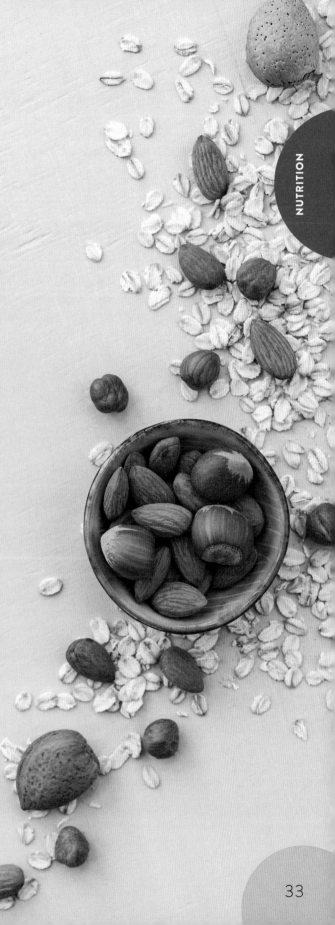

coeliac disease. For those with coeliac disease, eating gluten causes the body to attack the villi (the tiny finger-like projections in the intestines that absorb nutrients from food). Thus their ability to absorb nutrients is compromised and this leads to nutritional deficiencies of, for example, iron and vitamins D and B12.

Those who have non-coeliac gluten sensitivity do *not* tend to develop the nutrient deficiencies commonly seen in coeliacs. They do, however, have a higher tendency to get skin irritations and inflammation. Research has found that more than half of patients with non-coeliac gluten sensitivity also presented with hives and swelling (36 per cent), generalised itching (10 per cent), psoriasis (nine per cent) and eczema (45 per cent). The good news is that, with a definite diagnosis of non-coeliac gluten sensitivity, they were able to resolve these problems by adopting a gluten-free diet.

Please note: it is very important to consult both your GP and an Accredited Practising Dietitian *before* considering the removal of gluten from your diet – gluten needs to be present in the body for a proper diagnosis to be made.

Food chemicals:
salicylates, amines & glutamate

Not everyone's skin problems are the same, nor are they triggered by the same foods. So keep reading before you rush to empty your pantry of every food containing wheat or gluten, corn, oat and soy that you can find.

When we hear the word 'chemical', we generally assume that means something unnatural, toxic, nasty and no good for us, like MSG, right? But some chemicals occur naturally in lots of healthy foods such as fruits, vegetables, meats, nuts and spices. These compounds are called salicylates, amines and glutamate and they can be used as natural additives to enhance flavour and freshness.

Some people are more sensitive than others to these natural chemicals and can experience adverse reactions: symptoms might include hives, rashes, eczema, dermatitis, headaches, stomach problems, feeling irritable and just feeling generally unwell or run down. The severity of the reaction depends on how much and which combinations of food chemicals are consumed. Each person has a different 'threshold' that their body can tolerate before they tip over into symptoms. This is why it's difficult to identify culprit foods when reactions can take hours, days or even weeks to build up to an individual's threshold.

Each person has a different 'threshold' that their body can tolerate before they tip over into symptoms.

● ● ●

SALICYLATES occur naturally in many fruits, vegetables, nuts, herbs and spices, jams, honey, yeast extracts, tea, coffee, juice, beer and wines. They are also found in products such as flavourings, perfumes, cosmetic products, oils such as pepper-mint and eucalyptus oil, and in some medications, such as aspirin.

AMINES are a result of fermentation, or a breaking down of proteins in food. Foods such as cheese, chocolate, yeast extract, wines, beer and fish products contain high concentrations of amines. They also occur in fruits and vegetables, such as bananas, avocados, tomatoes and some legumes.

GLUTAMATE is naturally found in the majority of foods we eat. Glutamate is often added to foods to enhance or strengthen the flavour; think of all your favourite meals that include tomatoes, cheese, mushrooms, stock cubes, sauces and meat or yeast extracts. It's the natural glutamate that you're tasting.

So, perhaps you've cut out processed food and the ingredients that commonly cause intolerances, such as wheat, dairy, nuts and eggs, and you're trying to eat healthily, but you still can't shake a feeling of perpetual fatigue, an unsettled stomach or perhaps unsightly rashes? It could be a naturally occurring food chemical in all that healthy food you're eating that is triggering your symptoms.

This is one of the reasons that being tested and getting professional help is so useful: you need not restrict your diet more narrowly than necessary. Instead, it is best to work with a dietitian to identify the true food issues, supervise an elimination diet, if needed, and help you to develop a balanced eating plan that will meet all your dietary requirements, while still incorporating a good variety of foods.

Hydration & alcohol

It is well known that alcohol dehydrates your body, including the skin, and this will happen every time you drink. We don't fully understand what it is in alcohol that causes dehydration: it produces excessive urination, but we're not sure why; it also reduces the amount of antidiuretic hormone you make. Even if you drink a lot of water, about half or two-thirds of it is urinated out, so you will still be dehydrated after drinking.

Dehydration can lead to fine lines and wrinkles on the skin, to irritation of blood vessels in the eyes, spider veins and enlarged red blood vessels in the face. Drinking in excess is also thought to deprive the skin of vital vitamins and nutrients; in particular, vitamin A and zinc. Rosacea, a skin disorder that starts with a tendency to blush and flush easily (the 'red-wine flush') can also lead to permanent changes, such as broken blood vessels and reddening.

Alcohol is calorie-dense: one gram of alcohol contains nearly the same amount of calories as one gram of fat, so it is calorie loaded, but with none of the nutrients. Drinking in excess can create bloated, puffy faces too.

The Australian government guidelines on alcohol consumption recommend that healthy adults should drink no more than two standard drinks on any day; however, the latest scientific research suggests that 10 standard drinks per week should be the limit. I would, however, suggest that if you really want great skin you shouldn't be having more than three or four standard drinks per week, sorry. If you are drinking alcohol, good advice is to drink a glass of water after each glass of alcohol: this will slow your alcohol consumption and keep you hydrated.

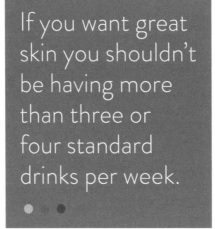

If you want great skin you shouldn't be having more than three or four standard drinks per week.

As we are taught at school, the human body is approximately 75 per cent fluid, and water has a key role in normal physiological balance. Water is the main component of human cells and tissues, including the skin. Cutaneous water content (water in the skin) is known to play an important role in different skin functions, especially as a protective barrier and defence against infection.

Recent research has shown that higher water content in your diet does positively impact normal skin physiology, in particular, hydration and intracellular behaviour. As a general rule, the Australian government advises we should aim for at least 2.5 litres of fluid per day — this can include tea, coffee, plain mineral water and soda water — but keep in mind that these can contain sodium, and, of course, caffeine, which should be consumed in moderation.

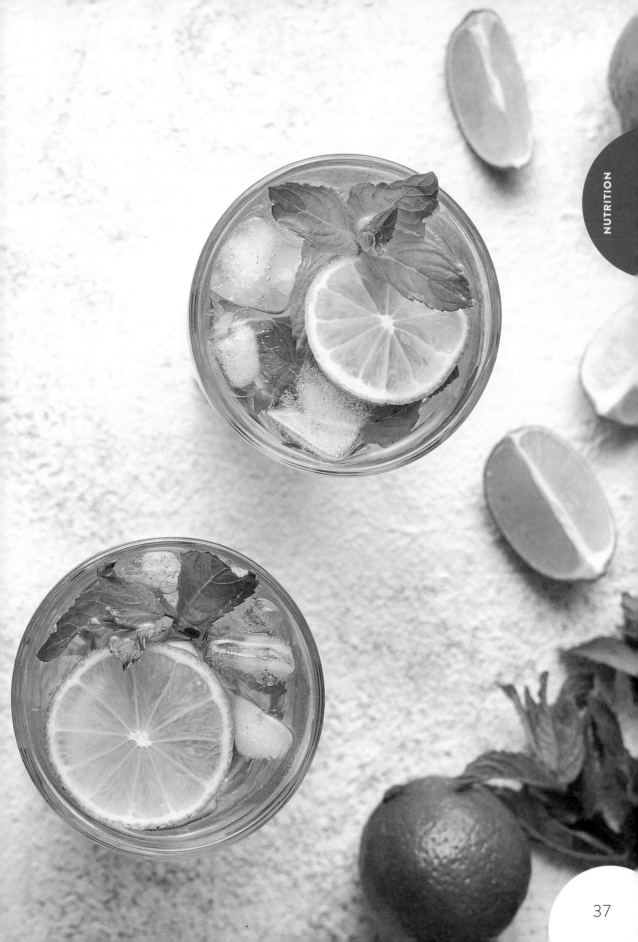

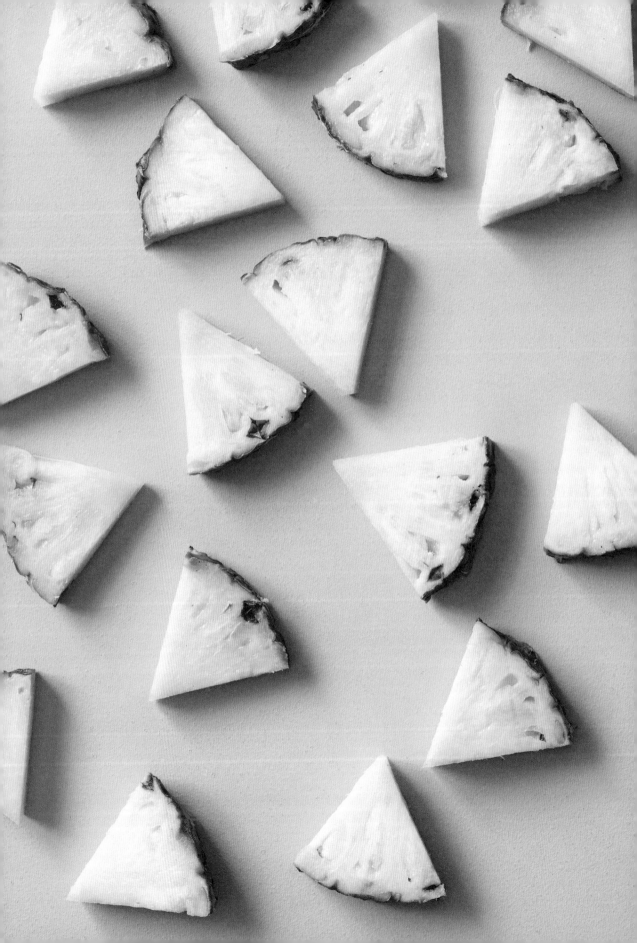

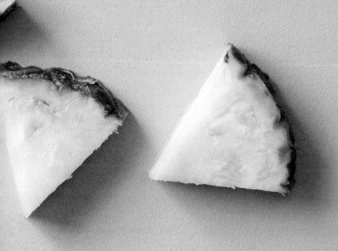

CHAPTER 3

GUT HEALTH AND YOUR SKIN

WELCOME TO THE MICROBIOME

Italian gastroenterologist Dr Alessio Fasano said, rather fabulously, in 2010: 'The gut is not Las Vegas. What happens in the gut does not stay in the gut.' In fact, there is a growing body of evidence to show that the gut is the axis on which the rest of our health pivots.

Our gastrointestinal tract (gut) is the tubing along which food travels between stomach and rectum. The main function of the gut is to absorb nutrients from food and expel what the body doesn't need. The gut is populated by trillions of bacterial microorganisms that regulate digestion, immune function, hormone production and much more. These microorganisms collectively are known as the gut microbiome; we are learning more and more about how the microbiome affects all the workings of the body, including the health of the skin. When the microbiome isn't working well, this can lead to diarrhoea or constipation and nutrients not being properly absorbed by the gut, so they can reach other areas of the body (such as the skin) to bring nourishment.

Welcome to the gut–skin axis. Unlike the gut, which is in a constant state of flux, the skin performs its functions most effectively in a state of homeostasis or harmony. By managing our diet so that it feeds the right balance of good and bad bacteria in the gut, we are enabling a cascade of signals that supports healthy skin. If someone has a history of frequent antibiotic usage (which kill good bacteria in the gut, as well as the harmful bacteria they are targeting), low immunity, chronic dieting, restriction of certain food groups or not eating enough fibre, some of the healthy bacteria in their gut can be starved. And that will show up in the skin.

The gut microbiome is constantly changing and it needs fuel to multiply and rejuvenate. It is fed by carbohydrates and fibre (soluble and insoluble), from foods such as oats, beans and legumes.

We're living in the era of sanitisation, when no germ is safe from antibacterial hand wipes and foaming cleansers, and some people find it a confronting thought that bacteria are living on every millimetre of our skin. There is an intimate relationship between the skin and gut microbiome, both influenced by the environment we live in and by each other. The 'microbial habitats' we create and what we put into our bodies are of equal importance. Lifestyle — such as extreme diets or cutting out certain foods — and medications — such as antibiotics — can wipe out certain bacteria from our gut: a counterproductive response that strips away the natural barrier of friendly bacteria and allows bad bacteria to overpopulate. Being exposed to natural microbial environments can promote a healthy balance of bacteria, both in our gut and on our skin.

WHY POTATO ISN'T 'BAD'

Potato (not just the skin, the flesh too) is a great source of resistant starch. Our bodies can't break that resistant starch down until it reaches the gut microbiome, which works to break it down into butyrate. Butyrate has been found to be great for our health and even 'cancer resistant'. Increased butyrate can promote a healthy microbiome, an excellent cycle of good health.

Inflammation

What happens if your gut microbiome is not balanced, or 'in biosis'? Essentially, this leads to inflammation, an often overused and misunderstood term to describe 'dysbiosis' (lack of balance), which can lead to disease. Dysbiosis has been linked to allergies, eczema and autoimmune disorders, as well as inflammatory skin conditions such as psoriasis, rosacea and acne. Although, it's a bit of a chicken-and-egg situation, in that we don't know for certain whether dysbiosis causes disease or disease causes dysbiosis, we *do* know that where you find one, you'll find the other. For example, people with rosacea are more likely to also have Crohn's disease, coeliac disease, small intestinal bacterial overgrowth (SIBO), irritable bowel syndrome (IBS) or *Helicobacter pylori* (the bacteria responsible for stomach ulcers, among other things). Those with dermatitis herpetiformis can even experience the same intestinal damage from eating gluten as someone with coeliac disease.

IRRITABLE BOWEL SYNDROME

This can manifest as many different symptoms such as abdominal pain, discomfort, wind, irregular bowel motions, bloating, diarrhoea or constipation. Skin can be affected by all of these: if you have diarrhoea, your gut will not be digesting nutrients properly and that will show up on your skin. There is a higher incidence of skin problems, such as eczema, in people suffering with IBS.

Leaky gut?

Feeling bloated? You might want to blame leaky gut. Headaches and tired? That too can be leaky gut. Brain fog? Leaky gut. Feeling irritable? Leaky gut. Leaky gut is the new Irritable Bowel Syndrome. Leaky gut really can be the explanation for all manner of ailments. Think of your stomach as a bucket of water: if it has holes in it, you're not going to get very far, but you might not realise anything until it's too late.

The layer of cells lining your small intestine absorbs nutrients from the food you eat. If you have leaky gut, undigested proteins can leak through the gut wall and into the bloodstream. Inflammation, gut dysbiosis, stress and toxic overload can all cause this 'intestinal permeability'. Your immune system then sends out signals to attack the 'foreign' food particles with antibodies. This is the theory behind food allergies and intolerances, and why people might develop one or two to begin with, but then become seemingly allergic to many foods they've eaten for years with no problem. Their immune system has gone into overdrive to 'protect' them from the foreign particles that are leaking through the gut wall, increasing inflammation in the body. Consequently, they might experience headaches, fatigue, bloating, diarrhoea, constipation, gas, nutritional deficiencies and a poor immune system, leading to frequent colds and illness. These can all be very vague symptoms to diagnose. There is, however, convincing evidence to suggest that prebiotics, probiotics and zinc can reduce inflammation and help restore intestinal permeability.

Probiotics: one bug does not fit all

Probiotics are live bacteria taken as an oral supplement, to provide a beneficial effect on your gut microbiome by increasing the number and variety of good bacteria. We are starting to learn that your gut bacteria rule your world; when they change or are out of balance, they affect the ability of the lining of the gut to absorb nutrients, which in turn affects your weight, your mental health, your energy and your skin. So it's no wonder that we have put so much hope in probiotics. Manufacturers promise that these magical pills are the key to health and vitality. But, if we put everything else aside, do they deliver when it comes to skin?

Unfortunately, one bug does *not* fit all. There are different bacterial strains, different 'strengths' and different dosage recommendations, variations in quality and an overwhelmingly increasing number of products to choose from on the probiotic market. And how are you meant to know if you even need a probiotic? Or which one is right for you? Or whether these probiotics are really going to improve your general health, let alone your skin concerns?

Everyone's gut and skin microbiome is individual, and we all have unique needs. We already know the ways in which healthy bacteria could have been starved; similarly, if someone has a parasite, a fungal infection or harmful bacterial overgrowth in their gut, this too will need to be considered when selecting the right probiotic and eating plan.

There is no blanket rule or single product that is 'best'. People should approach probiotics in the same way they would approach rehabilitation after a sporting injury, for example. You would get an assessment from a physiotherapist to identify the problem that is causing you pain, and then they'd recommend particular exercises to fix your specific problem. You wouldn't go off and just make up your own rehab plan, right? Arguably, probiotics require the same expert input and guidance to ensure that you are taking the right

Approach probiotics the same way you would approach rehabilitation after a sporting injury.

● ● ●

product for your needs. It's about the *ratios* of various species rather than the number of bacteria in our gut (so more does not equal better).

Some people could do more harm than good by buying a random probiotic off the shelf, or adding a whole lot of fermented prebiotic foods to their diet all at once. This could only worsen the problem, causing more bloating, gas, diarrhoea and skin problems and so on: all the things they were trying to fix in the first place. Having said that, different strains of bacteria do appear to have benefits for different conditions. Some studies have found probiotics to have beneficial effects on psoriasis, dermatitis and acne, thanks to their anti-

inflammatory, antimicrobial and immune system–modulating effects.

Lactobacillus and *Bifidobacterium* strains of bacteria appear to have a beneficial anti-inflammatory effect on skin cells. They also play a role in leaky gut syndrome by reducing inflammation and strengthening the mucosal barrier. There is even some limited research to suggest that applying *Lactobacillus* in topical formulations directly onto the skin might help restore a healthy skin microbiome.

These are two very common strains of gut-friendly bacteria used in commercial products. Dosage recommendations vary, but 5 to 10 million 'colony-forming units' (CFUs) in children and 10 to 20 million CFUs in adults is an adequate dose to support general health in most people.

Different strains of probiotic can be used to target different skin conditions; *L. acidophilus* and *bulgaricus* are recommended for acne; *rhamnosus* for UV skin damage; *reuteri, delbrueckii* and *salivarius* for atopic dermatitis. However, it is best to consult a healthcare professional to devise a plan for your personal needs before you start taking regular probiotics.

FERMENTED FOODS

While we're on the subject of probiotics, we must talk about the buzzword on every modern menu. Fermented foods have become the secret elixir to fix all ailments according to #instafood #happytummies #guthealth. But are they just #expensivemould?

Fermented foods have gained traction in recent years as a natural source of probiotics, which have been shown to help improve certain skin conditions. But this isn't a green light to eat all the fermented foods you can get your hands on. For a few reasons: just as with probiotic supplements, different skin conditions might benefit from different strains of bacteria and there is no such thing as a one-bug-fits-all approach. Secondly, somewhere along the way we've forgotten that, like any other therapeutic treatment, fermented foods should be eaten in medicinal, therapeutic amounts. It can be a fun weekend project to try your hand at fermenting your own vegetables, but you need to be very careful that jars are thoroughly sterilised and you follow all instructions in the recipes. There are plenty of cookbooks and internet instructions available.

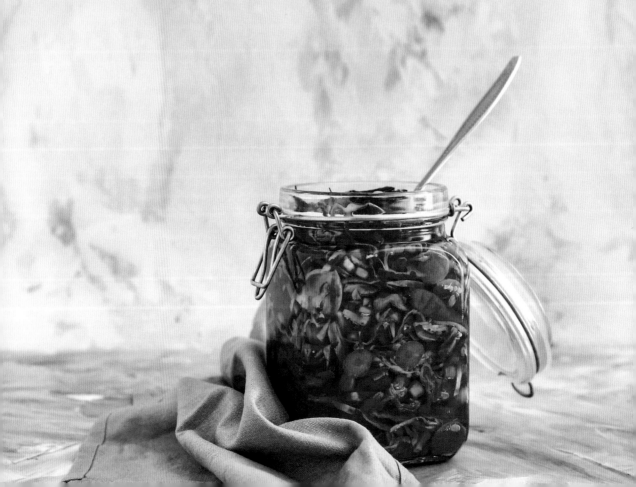

Prebiotics: you are what your gut bugs eat

Let's face it, it's not until you reach a ripe old age that you realise how much fibre makes your world go round. But if you thought fibre was one-dimensional, think again. Prebiotics are a type of non-digestible fibre that comes from vegetables, particularly starchy vegetables, fruit, legumes and wholegrains. These are fermented in the gut, producing a short-chain fatty acid, called butyrate, which feeds the good bacteria (probiotics), stimulates mucus production, reduces the intestinal permeability that results in leaky gut, and reduces inflammation. So, in simple, everyday terms, what does this mean you should eat? A healthy, sustainable, 'balanced' diet that includes adequate fibre from fresh vegetables, fruit, legumes and wholegrains.

It might sound tempting to eat low-carb, grain-free, gluten-free, or any other fad diet that promises a 'quick fix' or fast weight loss. But ultimately these shortcuts will only hinder your long-term progress, and they could worsen the state of your gut microbiome and therefore your skin health without you even realising it. The good news is, the more we find out about gut health and its impact on skin, the more we know about how to target specific skin conditions via nutrition. Learning how to eat for your microbiome will get you looking and feeling great, both inside and out, by working *with* your body, not against it.

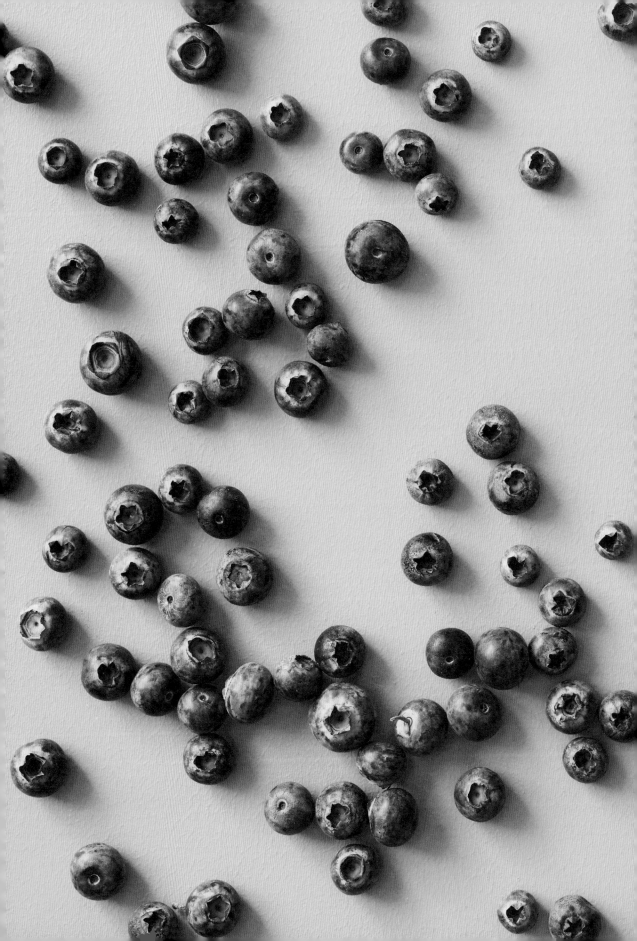

CHAPTER 4

SKIN HEALTH: COMMON CONDITIONS

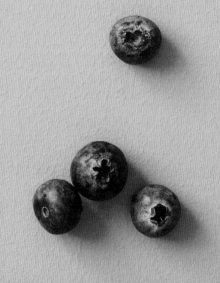

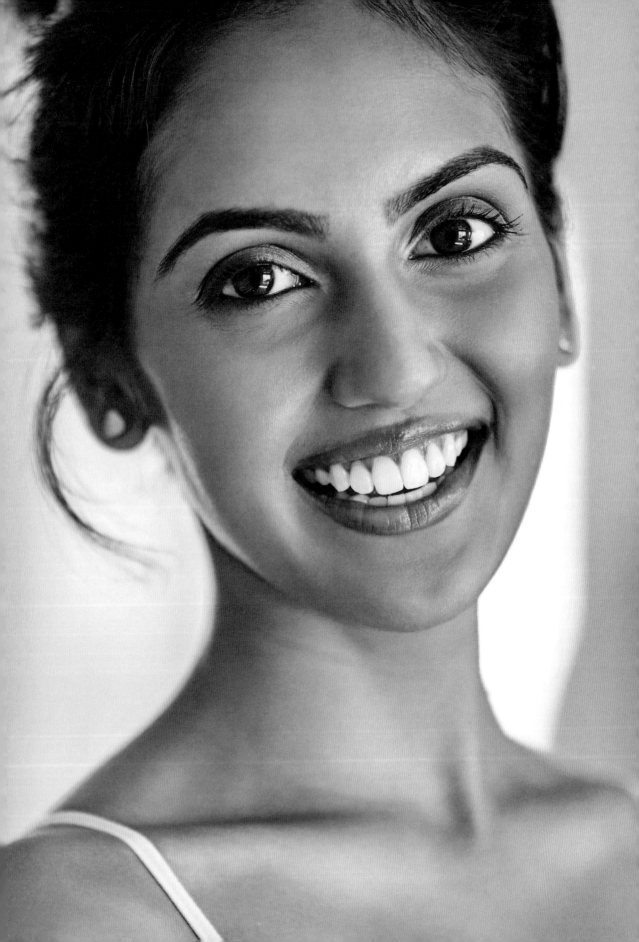

GETTING A DIAGNOSIS

Knowledge of skin health and common conditions will help you understand the role of dietary support and what you should cat, while working with your medical team. I've helped my patients overcome some common skin conditions — rashes, acne and psoriasis — by using targeted nutritional approaches. The first step is to get the right diagnosis, which will help your dermatologist determine the correct treatment options, and then to follow up with the best dietary and nutritional guidance and support.

PSORIASIS:
Flaky, angry, inflamed skin

There's no mistaking the red, dry and scaly patches of psoriasis. 'Flaky, angry skin, and no moisturiser works,' is the common complaint. It's a miserable, chronic inflammation disease that affects people's sleep, work and confidence.

Anyone who's had psoriasis knows the insatiable itch it can cause and the despair of unsightly patches that can show up anywhere. It's commonly seen on the knees, elbows, lower back, legs, stomach and sometimes under the armpits or on the scalp. Around half of all people with psoriasis will experience thickening of their nails and yellow oil spots on their nails. There are different types of psoriasis, which should be diagnosed by a doctor or dermatologist.

Why is psoriasis so common? It all comes down to inflammation. Inflammation inhibits normal physiology and homeostasis of skin cells, leading to conditions such as psoriasis, which point to deeper metabolic turmoil. Like many skin conditions, psoriasis is a combination of genetics, a hyperactive immune system and environmental stressors, which is what makes it so hard to control. If you've ever experienced trauma, emotional stress, change in climate, an infection, struggled with weight or taken certain medications, you might have experienced a flare-up of psoriasis, but never made the connection.

Another probable culprit that's not so well known is insulin resistance. When the body is in a state of chronic inflammation, this inhibits the signalling pathway of insulin, causing insulin resistance. As a result, the insulin is not as effective at moving sugar out of the bloodstream to the body's cells. The pancreas responds by producing progressively greater amounts of insulin and can eventually wear itself out, leading to type 2 diabetes.

Something else that can cause inflammation is immune health, including non-coeliac gluten sensitivity. While this diagnosis doesn't lead to intestinal damage from eating wheat, as someone with coeliac disease would experience, it can manifest as itchy skin rashes such as psoriasis. So what are the treatment options? These are some of the options you could easily try.

LIFESTYLE If you're serious about improving your health and skin, smoking and drinking need to go. If you are already battling psoriasis, then toxins such as nicotine and alcohol put unnecessary strain on your body to process and eliminate them. Meditation and acupuncture might help improve psoriasis as well, by reducing stress — stress has been shown to trigger psoriasis flare-ups in emotional times.

MEDICATION Because an overactive immune system can lead to psoriasis, the first line of treatment is usually topical steroid creams or ointments: these are very effective in suppressing the body's acute inflammatory response, which in turn reduces the symptoms. But this is not a long-term solution. Some people can experience a 'rebound effect' after finishing the treatment, when their symptoms return worse than before, especially if they have not made positive lifestyle changes.

A traditional Chinese herb called indigo naturalis (Qing Dai), often used as a topical treatment for skin and nails, has shown scientific evidence in improving psoriasis; however, such remedies should never be used as a substitute for medical advice.

Inflammation caused by the immune system can be treated with biological agents. These drugs, made of organic material — human, plant, animal or microbe — dampen the immune response.

NUTRITION There's some speculation about turmeric and its anti-inflammatory health benefits; in the case of psoriasis

there is truth behind this. Curcumin, the active ingredient in turmeric, has been shown to reduce dryness, redness and the thickness of psoriasis plaques, either as a topical or oral formulation.

If you have been diagnosed with insulin resistance, it's important to manage it with your doctor and an Accredited Practising Dietitian, as certain medications and a low-GI balanced eating plan can prevent further progression of this problem. This can also, importantly, improve skin integrity. The Mediterranean diet has also been found to be helpful, due to its well-known anti-inflammatory effects. This is particularly due to the omega-3s and monounsaturated fats found in extra virgin olive oil, fish, seafood and nuts. A diet rich in vegetables and legumes is also effective. Supplementing with fish oil on its own has less evidence to support its effectiveness than the Mediterranean diet.

If you have had a positive blood test and medical diagnosis for non-coeliac gluten sensitivity or coeliac disease, a 100 per cent gluten-free diet might help reduce symptoms of psoriasis, but this is for a small minority of people and should be managed by your healthcare experts.

Due to the role of vitamin D in skin-barrier maintenance and immunity, vitamin D deficiency is also associated with a higher risk of psoriasis. In this case, supplementation may assist. Some psoriasis patients have also reported improvements after avoiding nightshade vegetables, such as eggplant, tomato and white potato, as well as processed sugar.

PSORIASIS
KAREN

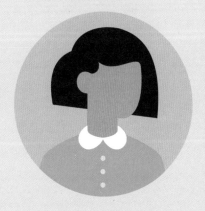

By the time Karen turned 50 years old she had been through a long battle with her health. It had started with endometriosis when she was young, followed by ovarian cancer at 48 years old. Around that same time she started experiencing very dry, scaly, inflamed skin on her hands, which exacerbated her feelings of stress and anxiety. For two years Karen endured the worsening psoriasis until she made the decision that she needed help.

CAUSES

Reaching out to an expert dermatologist, and using topical creams and biological agents, helped to alleviate the acute symptoms of Karen's psoriasis, but it was not until the dermatologist dug deeper that they discovered an underlying insulin resistance. Karen was then referred to me to provide nutritional therapy that would go below the skin and address the true cause of her systemic health problems, rather than treating the symptoms only.

It became apparent that insulin resistance was a primary cause of her psoriasis and was creating her skin inflammation. This also explained Karen's fluctuating weight, particularly during treatment for ovarian cancer, which exacerbated her underlying metabolic disease. For Karen, dealing with psoriasis in such a visual area — her hands

— and battling constant fatigue was a really challenging experience in her demanding job, where there were high expectations of performance and presentation.

TRIGGERS

It's clear that stress was a major trigger for Karen. The stress of coping with her ovarian cancer treatment exacerbated her psoriasis and day-to-day stresses. The pressure of maintaining the responsibilities of her job in a management role and doing shiftwork was clearly starting to show. Missing meals played a big role — she ate small amounts during the day and overate at night, often takeaway foods that are high in sugar, high in fat and with a high GI. Such calorie-dense foods can exacerbate weight gain and insulin resistance and hence trigger symptoms. And so it becomes a vicious cycle.

NUTRITION

We kept the plan simple and easy to achieve. For Karen the focus was on a balanced diet of foods that were grab-and-go to fit her busy schedule. Meals focused on low-GI carbohydrates, balanced protein and good fats that were satiating so she felt full and happy throughout the day and would be able to maintain a good eating pattern. It was important for her to not miss meals and to establish a routine pattern of eating. We focused on foods that didn't spike insulin production and would promote constant energy so that Karen avoided reaching for caffeine, soft drinks or sugary snacks to get through the day.

RESULT

A tailored meal plan helped Karen plan her days with interesting food that kept her full and happy. It was important to establish her carbohydrate threshold — so Karen understood how much carbohydrate her body could tolerate without triggering increased insulin production. Initially she was very scared about which foods she could eat and, rather than creating a whole list of foods she had to avoid, we were able to simplify that. Wholegrain, low-GI bread was still allowed, and a sandwich of good protein was something she could have that would improve her overall health outcome.

Together with her biological-agent medications and other medications for her metabolic health, by creating a meal plan of food she could easily follow, Karen's skin very much improved in a matter of three to four weeks. This was very motivating for Karen to continue.

Other benefits came hand in hand, such as higher energy levels, weight loss without feeling that she was dieting, and a regular pattern of eating. We also made sure to rule out any other complications, such as anaemia, and supplemented her vitamin D deficiency as well.

The best part was that we simplified the message for Karen so that it was sustainable in the long term, combined with her busy lifestyle and work demands.

ACNE :
Adolescence is just
one big walking pimple

Acne has long been the punchline of jokes about teenagers, but it's nothing to laugh about. After all, it affects a whopping 90 per cent of adolescents in Western societies. Anyone who's ever experienced acne will know how emotionally isolating and shattering it can be for a person's self-confidence. Many of my patients express feeling dirty, or hopeless because they don't know what else to do when products don't work. Advertising often oversimplifies acne treatment, building false hope and confusing those who suffer from it. In reality, it takes an incredible amount of trust in the process.

Firstly, is must be made clear that acne has nothing to do with being unclean; it is a normal part of hormonal changes during puberty. In both males and females, testosterone levels rise which, in turn, signals to the skin to increase oil (sebum) production. This can cause hair follicles to become blocked or clogged with oil or an overgrowth of bacteria, which then becomes inflamed and manifests itself as those unsightly blackheads or whiteheads.

Acne most commonly occurs on the face, neck, back and chest as the sebaceous glands are the largest and most active in these areas. Acne might show itself as a combination of whiteheads, blackheads, pustules, papules, cysts or nodules. What's the difference?

Whiteheads are usually small white raised bumps under the skin, whereas blackheads are often flat, with a dark keratin plug in the centre. Pustules are what you might envisage when you think of a 'pimple': a raised pus-filled bump that might range from 2 mm to 5 mm across. Papules or nodules are commonly referred to as 'hormonal acne'. This kind of acne appears as firm, red, inflamed spots and lesions on the skin. Breakouts often occur along the jawline, chin and neck area; they are painful and can leave permanent scarring.

LIFESTYLE The truth is that hormonal changes are only part of the picture. Adolescent angst isn't without reason: this is a period of great change and flux in a person's body, relationships, emotions, lifestyle, academic stress and diet. It's a hard enough time of life without also having to deal with acne and the social stigma that comes with it.

Many teens become less physically active during their high school years and lose interest in Mum's packed lunch when they suddenly catch sight of the school canteen. And, while many parents don't want to hear it, the reality is that around 40 per cent of teens aged 14 years and over in Australia regularly consume alcohol. Surging hormones, physical inactivity, junk food, alcohol, not enough sleep, stress, make-up and sometimes improper skin care ... all this combined with excessive oil production becomes the perfect storm.

MEDICATION There are many different lotions, potions and pills for acne and usually it's a process of trial and error to see what works for you. Retinoids, salicylic acid or benzoyl peroxide are often used in topical washes and creams to reduce the amount of bacteria on the skin, and to encourage repair, growth and hydration. Low-dose antibiotics can help reduce bacterial overgrowth; or, for girls, the contraceptive pill might be used to reduce the amount of testosterone in the body if that is causing abnormal oil production. In more severe cases, medications are used that may have more systemic effects on the body, and the side effects might include skin dryness, peeling, redness, irritation and cardiovascular complications.

Depending on the cause of the acne, many of these treatments can provide relief of symptoms, but often are just a temporary fix for a deeper metabolic dysfunction. When treatment stops, acne often comes back with a vengeance.

NUTRITION So, what does metabolic dysfunction have to do with acne? Once again, it's inflammation. It's true for everyone that steady insulin levels ensure our body is functioning optimally, but this is especially true for many people with skin conditions. This was shown in a Melbourne study that found that a low-GI diet significantly reduced insulin sensitivity and acne. This study supports a growing body of research that says well-balanced nutrition with adequate protein, low-GI carbohydrates and healthy fats should be at the centre of treatment. Zinc supplements might also help improve the symptoms of acne.

Dairy is often a sensitive topic when it comes to skin, but don't be too quick to discount it. Dairy milk consumption has been linked to the presence of acne, regardless of whether it was low-fat, skim or full-fat; however, yoghurt and cheese are not associated with acne. But if you enjoy dairy, don't be alarmed. Many people are fine with dairy and don't need to remove it from their diets. If you are recommended to reduce or remove dairy, it's important to consult an Accredited Practising Dietitian to ensure you are receiving enough nutrients from other foods to counteract this.

CASE STUDY
ACNE
TAYLOR

Taylor was an athlete, diagnosed with teenage acne by the time she was 16 years old. As a sprinter, she needed to maintain lean muscle mass, but suddenly she was noticing changes in her weight. I was very mindful that teenagers have to 'grow into their skin': it's important that we look at their growth and development, and that it's not a reflection on them personally. At that time in life there are hormonal changes, self-esteem struggles, skin problems, weight fluctuation and going through high school. All are factors that we have to consider.

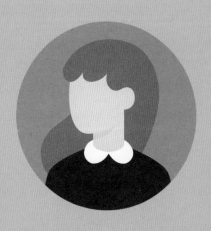

SYMPTOMS

Taylor was dealing with consistent pimples on her face, blackheads she was tempted to squeeze, and raised and inflamed lumps on her face, chest and shoulders. Taylor was insulin resistant, but didn't present as a typical insulin-resistant person because she was quite slim. I had to understand her activity levels, help her fuel her body for her running, and understand how acne and hormones interact so I didn't affect her performance in her sprint running.

TRIGGERS

When she experienced stress in her sport and school exams, Taylor's symptoms flared up. She also had low iron levels, which needed addressing. I had to work out her pattern of eating — the case with all my patients — but I also had to introduce nutrition principles. Research shows that highly processed foods in a teenage diet exacerbate skin problems and can inhibit wound healing. Because Taylor was a sprinter, she was always looking for refined carbohydrate foods as fuel during races, which unfortunately was triggering her acne. I had to figure out how this high level of fuel could be incorporated into her diet, as well as looking after her skin, alongside her dermatologist.

High insulin levels can cause glucose levels to go up and down, resulting in reactive hypoglycaemia. Taylor would feel shaky, tired, have sugar cravings and feel desperate to eat, leading to bingeing episodes and running out of fuel. On top of this, she was taking antibiotics for the acne and medication for her insulin resistance. So it was important I adjusted her food to make sure she had an even distribution of fuel, to avoid feeling so hungry that she felt a loss of control. Because insulin is linked to the hormones that produce acne, we introduced low-GI carbohydrates at each meal, balanced with protein and good fats, to lower the insulin response.

In addition, Taylor had increased iron requirements due to her sport and menstruation, so we had to ensure she had enough iron in her diet too. Often when teenagers crave sugar, it can be due to low iron. So, correcting that deficiency really helped with her sugar habits.

NUTRITION

Taylor's endocrine disturbance was managed by medication and a nutritional component. Our main nutritional focus was in finding food swaps — such as liquid meals, smoothies and snacks — for training days and race days. These had to be low GI, with balanced protein and good fats, such as apples with nuts, crackers with cheese, or basmati rice with lean chicken, instead of chips. I concentrated on balancing her snacking.

RESULT

By focusing on food swaps, we ensured that Taylor still felt 'light' before a race without any nausea during competitions. Not only was she achieving better times in her races, but she also had more energy, faster recovery times and her skin was much improved. We also had to be mindful of her race weight, so we had to work out both her diet for the off-season and running season. She is now studying overseas on a university sports scholarship.

OILY SKIN & POLYCYSTIC OVARIES :
The second adolescence?

This section is for all the ladies out there who feel at war with their own bodies. Whoever said self-love and gratitude are the secret to happiness clearly has never had polycystic ovary syndrome (PCOS).

This is a complex metabolic and hormonal condition that affects 20 per cent of women, who also often struggle with insulin resistance. It's often a shock for women who suddenly develop issues with acne and excessive body hair on their face and body (hirsutism), which can be among the first signs of hormonal imbalance. These imbalances can also lead to amenorrhoea (absence of periods), irregular or painful periods, infertility and struggles with weight. Some women can experience oily or thinning hair on their head too.

LIFESTYLE Many women tend to ignore changes happening in their bodies and skin, because hormones are a fact of life. But it's important to know what's normal and when to see a doctor. Diagnosing PCOS early on can also help identify the insulin resistance that can be associated with the condition; however, the reality is that many women with PCOS and insulin resistance remain undiagnosed, as doctors may be more inclined to identify the condition in those who are overweight or obese, despite the fact that around half of women with PCOS and insulin resistance are underweight or healthy weight. The risk is that, if undetected, insulin resistance increases the risk of developing type 2 diabetes, metabolic disease and even obesity. Women are told to go away and eat properly and exercise to lose some weight, the implication being that this is self-inflicted, which leads to feelings of guilt. It's hard enough for many women to like what they see in the mirror without dealing with a condition like PCOS as well. It's no wonder, then, that poor self-esteem, disordered eating, depression and low libido can result.

The good news for people who are struggling with acne, excess hair and body image problems is that these can be corrected after they are diagnosed with PCOS. As part of the diagnosis, hormone levels will be tested — in particular, androgens (male hormones), thyroid function, prolactin and follicle-stimulating hormone (FSH). Most of which can be corrected so that the body and skin can begin to function normally again.

MEDICATION As well as preventing conception, oral contraceptives ('the pill') are a common and effective treatment for PCOS and often result in clearer skin. They reduce ovarian male hormone secretion, which usually improves acne and excess body hair, as well as regulating the menstrual cycle. This can provide great relief for women who experience erratic and prolonged bleeding.

But what happens when you go off the pill? Situations change, and what was right for you at one point in your life might not be right for you now. Going on or off contraception is a personal decision; for example, it might no longer be needed if you're thinking about starting a family. But what often happens is these women struggle to establish a regular cycle, their skin begins to break out again and the symptoms of PCOS creep back into the picture. They can feel as if they're back at square one. This is often because the underlying problem — insulin resistance — is still driving the side effects of systemic inflammation and hormonal imbalance.

Testing for insulin resistance should be carried out in all patients who suspect PCOS, not just overweight women. This involves two tests: one for fasting glucose and insulin, and a two-hour oral glucose tolerance test which shows how well insulin is working in the body.

If insulin resistance is diagnosed, there are things you can do to help yourself. Metformin is a drug often prescribed to regulate blood glucose and insulin levels. It has been shown to be effective in treating PCOS by restoring ovulation and a regular monthly cycle as well as supporting weight loss and reducing acne and hirsutism. It is considered a safe medication, with only slight gastrointestinal side effects.

NUTRITION It's probably no surprise that diet and exercise are crucial when it comes to managing PCOS and insulin resistance. Processed carbohydrates and refined sugar should be avoided and replaced with unprocessed low-GI carbs, healthy fats and adequate, balanced, lean protein. This will help keep insulin levels steady.

Resistance training is another secret weapon: not only does it help with fat loss and maintaining lean muscle, but it also reduces excess male hormone production and increases the levels of reproductive hormones in women.

There is limited evidence that a herbal extract of *Vitex agnus-castus*, might be effective in restoring regular menstrual cycles in some women with PCOS. There are only a small number of studies exploring the efficacy, therapeutic dosage and long-term effects of this natural plant-derived supplement, so approach with caution; however, generally no side effects are reported and it is likely safe when taken according to recommended dosage for short periods. It might also go by other names, such as chasteberry or vitagnus among other similar variations.

CASE STUDY

POLYCYSTIC OVARIES

MICHELLE

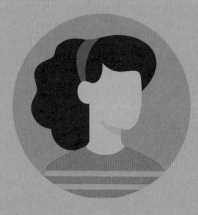

Michelle was 22 years old when she was diagnosed with polycystic ovaries and insulin resistance. She had been working with an endocrinologist prior to coming to see me, but hadn't ever had a dietitian go through her diagnosis and provide a plan. Michelle works as a personal trainer, is an avid sports woman, surf lifesaver and PE teacher and felt that she 'should know better'. Along with this came feelings of guilt because she couldn't lose weight, despite all her efforts, and she was embarrassed and frustrated. Because of the high levels of testosterone in her blood she put on muscle easily and eventually started feeling extremely masculine.

SYMPTOMS

When I met Michelle she'd been struggling for years with pimples, oily hair, oily skin, irregular periods and easy weight gain. She had tried all the fad diets — intermittent fasting, no carbs, yes: carbs, missing meals — even vegetarianism, to no avail.

Michelle is a young adult, but the social situations, binge drinking and eating out that seemed normal to her friends were all sabotaging her health. When she came to me she couldn't see a way out.

There is a misconception about insulin resistance that if you go away and 'just' eat properly and lose weight, it will fix the issue. Michelle was exercising and in her mind she was eating properly, but she felt as if she still couldn't lose weight.

NUTRITION

Normalising food again was the big challenge of Michelle's treatment. She had to learn to trust food again and not feel fearful of eating things like bread, for example. We helped structure her eating by providing a plan that worked with her schedule and gave her the confidence to eat. We improved her breakfasts and made sure she had more balanced snacks on standby and didn't miss lunch, which is not conducive to losing weight. It was also important that she understood the physiology and consistency of medication. We were able to address Michelle's social life on weekends and reduce the binge drinking. She needed education on which snack foods were the best choices, in a way that didn't make her feel she was missing out.

RESULT

Michelle found that having a strategy for the weekend helped. She learned to pace herself, set a limit of no more than two standard alcoholic drinks in any one sitting, avoided high-sugar mixers and always ate a meal before going out. But, most importantly, she learned not to beat herself up. She was happy to finally know what to eat, how to choose from menus and have a pattern of eating established. It was important for her to understand the principles of low-GI carbohydrates, balanced protein and good fats at breakfast, morning tea, lunch, afternoon tea and dinner.

These changes resulted in longer-lasting energy, better mood, and feeling less 'hangry'. We taught her how to feel full and happy and she enjoyed the change. So, the eating plan quickly became part of her own habit rather than something she had to be told to do.

In the space of six weeks she'd lost four kilograms, but more importantly she'd lost centimetres and a good percentage of fat. This meant her insulin was being regulated, which was regulating the testosterone that was associated with her polycystic ovaries. Overall her skin improved, her weight was coming down, her skin was less oily and her menstruation cycle was more regular. She was getting back to her old self.

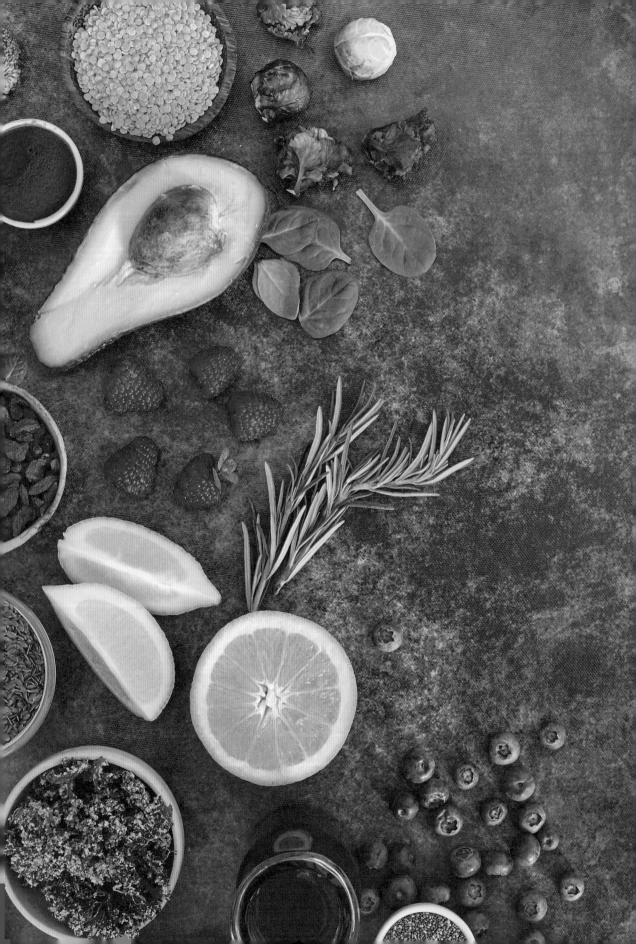

DERMATITIS HERPETIFORMIS:
The gluten rash

Hippocrates once said, 'All disease begins in the gut'. That didn't turn out to be quite true, but it is for dermatitis herpetiformis. This is a blistering autoimmune skin disease that usually affects more men than women, around the age of 30 to 40 years. There is a strong link between dermatitis herpetiformis and coeliac disease. Sufferers of both experience an intense autoimmune response after eating any food that contains gluten; both have Immunoglobulin A (IgA) antibodies, made by the immune system to fight antigens, such as bacteria or toxins, but in this case they fight the 'gluten' protein, found in wheat, rye, barley, oats and malt. They might both experience gastrointestinal symptoms, such as diarrhoea and stomach cramps, but those with dermatitis herpetiformis also develop blisters on the skin, due to inflammation caused by their autoimmune response. This usually develops around the elbows, knees, buttocks, scalp and neck.

Reversing dermatitis herpetiformis requires a lifelong 100 per cent gluten-free diet. As for people with coeliac disease, eating gluten causes intestinal damage to the villi in the small intestine. So it is vital that proper testing is done to prevent issues with malabsorption of nutrients. This involves a skin scraping of the blisters by a dermatologist and an endoscopy, by a gastroenterologist, to check for intestinal damage. Like any skin condition, a proper diagnosis makes for effective treatment. In this case, topical creams and medications help heal the skin by reducing inflammation and bacterial growth while the body takes time to respond to a gluten-free diet.

CASE STUDY

DERMATITIS

DAVID

David was 36 years old. As an accountant —
a 'systems man' — he doesn't like to be troubled by
many things. David had a chronic rash that had
bothered him for a long time, and he didn't know
why. He was referred to me by his gastroenterologist
because he was newly diagnosed with coeliac
disease, but I felt the coeliac disease was the
background to his unknowingly having a skin
condition called dermatitis herpetiformis.

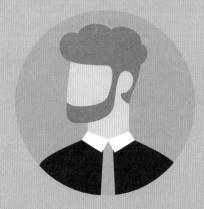

SYMPTOMS

David's rash was directly related to gluten
ingestion. David didn't even know he had
this, even though it had had a profound
impact on his life. He had thick scaly rashes
on both his knees and elbows, and it affected
the skin in his groin region so profoundly
that he eventually needed a skin graft. By
the time I saw him he had tried various
doctors and years of steroidal creams to
manage the itch, which had ruined his skin.
But no one had gone to the effort of further
investigation until now.

TREATMENT

Dermatitis herpetiformis is diagnosed by
skin biopsy; a dermatologist might order
antibody testing for coeliac disease and you
would be referred to a gastroenterologist.

To confirm the diagnosis, the gastroenterologist looks for signs of damage to
the villi on the surface of the small bowel.
Because David hadn't yet been diagnosed,
there had been quite a bit of damage done.

David had been taking sulfone in an
effort to reduce the swelling and control the
itchy rash on his skin caused by gluten
ingestion; however, the only effective
medical treatment for this condition is a
100 per cent gluten-free diet. But, because
David had been through so many
investigations, he couldn't believe that a
diet change was what was needed. He had
to really learn what going completely gluten
free meant and the impact that would have
on his skin. It was also hard for him to realise
that he couldn't go out and have a beer with
his mates.

NUTRITION

I taught David to understand where gluten is hidden and how to identify foods that contain it by reading ingredient lists, rather than relying on a manufacturer's 'gluten free' label to tell him which foods were safe to eat. Gluten is found in wheat, rye, barley, oats, malt and triticale. There is a great debate around oats — they can be purchased in the US as 'gluten free', but still contain avenin, a protein with similar amino-acid structure to gluten's gliadin. According to the Australian Coeliac Society, we don't know who will react to avenin.

Being confident at reading ingredient labels was a challenge for David. What about contamination? Would a bit of gluten do any harm? I took David on a shopping trip to help him understand how to read labels and decode ingredients, such as glucose syrup or caramel colour derived from wheat (which contains such minute amounts of gluten that it is technically gluten free).

RESULT

It took about three months for David to learn the skills required to eat a balanced gluten-free diet. This rid the gluten from his bloodstream and allowed his gut to mend so it wasn't triggering a rash. I had to teach David how to be prepared for contamination issues, to take food to work with him and be mindful when he ate out. A gluten-free pizza can't aways be guaranteed to be gluten free; it needs to be prepared in a safe gluten-free area and David needed to be confident enough to ask those questions.

David was very diligent about following the advice I gave him and he had a very good outcome. He controlled the itchy rash that had been plaguing him for years and was able to repair his gut and prevent long-term complications from coeliac disease.

HIVES & ECZEMA :
The insatiable itch

Hives — just the word makes me itchy. Hives don't discriminate: up to a quarter of people, young and old, will have hives at some stage in their life. Hives can last an hour or 24 hours (acute), or pop up intermittently over a long period of time (chronic). Either way, it feels like forever. Hives act like an allergic response, with sudden itchy, swollen, dry lesions or welts appearing.

Acute hives are often triggered by viral infection, some medications, food and other allergens, emotional stress and systemic diseases. Chronic hives are linked to autoimmune disorders, chronic infections such as hepatitis B and C, sinus infections and *Helicobacter pylori*. Around 35 to 40 per cent of cases of chronic hives are due to an autoimmune response, releasing histamines and pro-inflammatory molecules responsible for the itching.

Eczema comes from the Greek word meaning 'to boil'. It's often referred to as atopic dermatitis and as a childhood disease, as it develops during the first year of age, but adults can develop eczema too. Eczema appears as a scaly, crusty, red rash with moderate to severe itching. In adults it normally affects the sides of the neck, elbows, knees and hands with thickened dry patches. It's also common for the skin to become lightened or darkened post inflammation.

There are two types of eczema: atopic and non-atopic eczema. In atopic, high levels of antibodies will be found in the blood due to the body producing an autoimmune response to a food allergy. It often goes hand-in-hand with asthma and/or rhinitis, with 50 per cent of children with severe atopic eczema going on to develop asthma and 75 per cent developing allergic rhinitis. On the contrary, those with non-atopic will only show very low levels of antibodies. Non-atopic is more common in females and accounts for 10 to 45 per cent of cases. The cause of eczema is not yet fully understood; however, there are several factors that we know trigger or worsen the condition. Certain foods, environmental allergens, heat or cold, stress and genetics. Again, getting a medical diagnosis will support successful management, as the different types require different treatment protocols.

LIFESTYLE What do hives and eczema have in common? It is possible that both conditions may be caused by an underlying food allergy. First let's clarify the difference between an intolerance and an allergy.

Food allergies involve the immune system reacting to protein compounds in certain foods. Symptoms develop quickly, even immediately, or at least within a couple of hours after eating and may last a few hours or even several days. The symptoms of allergies can be life threatening.

Food intolerances don't involve the immune system at all. Reactions are dose dependent: a small amount is tolerable, but a large serving may trigger symptoms. Similarly, if the food is eaten regularly, there is a cumulative effect; for example, with small but daily exposure to the trigger food, it builds up in your system.

MEDICATION A regimen of antihistamine is often used to help gain control over a hives episode and offer symptomatic relief; however, in more than half of chronic hives cases, symptoms can last longer than 12 months. A long-term management strategy might use corticosteroids, such as Prednisone (though generally not as a first option: chances of rebound are high and side effects can be serious).

Most people with eczema use topical treatments (such as lotions, creams and ointments). It is very important to keep skin moisturised. Other supportive medications include topical immunomodulators which help with inflammation and are less likely to thin the skin. Antiseptic treatments, tar preparations, antibiotics, phototherapy and even non-steroidal immunosuppressants may also be used. Some people may need behavioural psychology support too. Speak with your medical team to work out the best treatment plan.

NUTRITION Food intolerances cause symptoms due to additives or chemicals naturally occurring in foods by irritating nerve endings. Some people are more sensitive than others and symptoms will vary.

There are several naturally occurring chemicals and additives that people might be sensitive to: salicylates, amines and glutamate (see pages 34–35 for more on these substances). These are found in many fresh foods such as fruits, vegetables, seasonings and nuts. They are also used as flavour and freshness enhancers. A good rule of thumb is the stronger the flavour, the higher the content of salicylates, amines and glutamates is likely to be.

If an allergen or irritant is identified, it's important to remove it so the individual is no longer exposed to the trigger. Foods that might be potential triggers in adults are shellfish, freshwater fish, berries, nuts, peanuts, pork, chocolate, tomatoes, spices, food additives and alcohol. In children, they tend to be milk, eggs, wheat, soy, seafood and nuts. It is important that food allergy testing is performed by a doctor so the culprit can be identified and removed from the diet without unnecessarily avoiding other nutritious foods.

CASE STUDY
ECZEMA
SAM

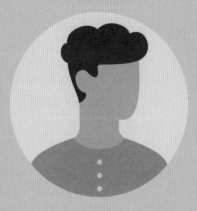

Sam is a 20-year-old very bright young man. He is a medical science university student who also spends a lot of time indoors playing computer games. He was increasingly tired, slept a lot and had unusual weight gain. Over the years Sam dealt with significant eczema, as well as asthma, but he didn't realise he had developed insulin resistance and a vitamin D deficiency.

SYMPTOMS

Sam's eczema had spread all over his face and body and was extremely itchy, which prevented him from getting a full night's sleep: he looked exhausted.

Sam's dermatologist referred him to me for nutritional support and by the time I met him, he was frustrated and fed up with symptoms that only seemed to worsen. He was considering dropping out of uni.

In the past Sam had tried a range of different topical creams plus UV therapy, and sometimes found relief, but it quickly reverted to acute symptoms. No one had thought about what he was eating.

TRIGGERS

On top of Sam's diet, I had to look at food chemicals and intolerances. You don't just get a reaction from the last food you ate, so it's hard to find triggers and patterns. It might not be until day three that you get a symptom and then you blame the last food you ate. As discussed earlier, salicylates, amines and glutamates are naturally occurring food chemicals and a lot of people forget that they're not actually chemicals that have been added to the food, but are found naturally in the food.

Knowing what chemicals are in foods can be simple. For example, does it contain lots of seeds, as in fruits like cucumbers and strawberries? Very colourful foods contain these chemicals. Dried fruits in particular contain such chemicals and then have sulphites added on top of that.

The allergy unit in Royal Prince Alfred Hospital offers an elimination diet, so we used a trigger journal to look at Sam's pattern of eating and to identify if there was a particular food chemical that he reacted to. Nitrates, found in ham and deli meats, were a key issue for Sam because he was eating them regularly. He would have bacon at breakfast and a ham sandwich at lunchtime; there would be a peak by the end of the week which resulted in exacerbation of his eczema.

NUTRITION

For Sam we had to address many different components that worked together. We lowered his food chemicals, supplemented his vitamin D and made sure any nutritional deficiencies were addressed. This was with a baseline low-GI, balanced protein and good fat eating plan. The hardest part for Sam was not to miss meals and mindlessly grab his default foods, which were high in the triggering chemicals.

RESULT

It took about six months for Sam to stop having flare-ups of his eczema, and then the dermatologist was able to decide what other treatments would be most beneficial.

71

ROSACEA :
The red wine flush

Rosacea is one of those skin problems that many people think they have. Their cheeks are always red and flushed, as if they've just come back from a run in the Arctic. Rosacea actually affects around 10 per cent of people and can be linked to genetics, sun exposure, pale skin tone, a type of mite (called *Demodex folliculorum*) and abnormal blood vessels of the face. But what many people don't know is that this is an inflammatory disorder. Those suffering from rosacea are more likely to have a problem with insulin resistance or gastrointestinal disorders, such as Crohn's disease, coeliac disease and *Helicobacter pylori*.

LIFESTYLE There are different kinds and varying severity of rosacea. Phymatous rosacea causes the skin around the nose to become thickened and nodular. Ocular rosacea causes redness, dryness, burning or stinging sensations on the eyelids and lower eye margins and is a precursor to facial rosacea, which normally presents as redness on the cheeks.

It is important to note that many people with rosacea have a history of topical steroid use, which is believed to contribute to the condition. They might also be sensitive to various face products, so it's strongly recommended that they discontinue using anything that causes irritation, including topical steroid products. Because rosacea is broken blood vessels close to the surface of the skin, exercise, hot or cold weather, emotional stress and topical steroids can increase the flushed appearance. Certain foods and drinks might also be triggers, such as alcohol, especially wine, hot beverages, spices and spicy food, sauces, any foods containing the food chemicals capsaicin (capsicum/peppers, chilli, paprika) or cinnamaldehyde (cinnamon, chocolate, citrus, tomatoes).

MEDICATION Most commonly, the treatment for rosacea is a course of low-dose antibiotics. To successfully treat rosacea, the triggers should be avoided and sun protection is a must. For some types of rosacea that are less responsive to antibiotics, intense pulsed light (IPL) and laser therapies might be more effective. Some doctors might prescribe topical antibiotic and retinoid creams. If the rosacea is linked to gastrointestinal problems, such as *Helicobacter pylori* or SIBO, antibiotics are extremely effective in inducing remission; however, antibiotics should always be used with caution, as regular use can lead to less biodiversity and changes in the composition of the gut microbiome, which might have implications for metabolic functioning and immunity.

NUTRITION Seeing that rosacea is, in part, an immune problem and correlates with various gut issues, sustained antibiotic use is unlikely to be helpful in the long run. As part of a long-term rosacea management and prevention strategy, proper nutrition is crucial for keeping metabolic, immune and gut health in order, which leads to healthy, well-nourished skin too. Other elements that could be beneficial for rosacea are including plenty of omega-3 fatty acids in the diet to help with inflammation. Potentially, zinc supplementation may also be beneficial in rosacea, as well as pre- and probiotics that support the immune system and gut functioning.

ROSACEA

MARY

Mary was nearing 60 years old and had never had any weight issues; she had always been lean, tall and slender. She was a hardworking, very organised, no-fuss woman, running her own business and doing a lot of bookwork. Mary was relatively healthy for her age, with a history of asthma and menopausal symptoms and some osteoarthritis.

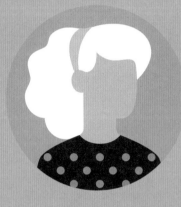

SYMPTOMS

All of a sudden Mary started putting on weight, experiencing irritable bowel symptoms and getting 'teenage' acne again. She had expected to be well and truly over that stage at 60 years old! When she started getting flushed in the face she assumed it must be linked to menopausal symptoms. Mary had gained 10 kilograms and was starting to feel very uncomfortable with the changes that were happening to her body.

TRIGGERS

As part of managing Mary's rosacea, I found there were foods that exacerbated her condition, such as hot beverages and alcohol. When she had a hot cup of tea or coffee or a few glasses of wine with friends she would start seeing more pimples and

look red and flushed in the face. She thought she must have an allergy to alcohol, but the alcohol itself was creating a trigger. Mary was also unknowingly eating capsaicin, found in spices and peppers and hot sauce, because she thought these were healthy for her metabolism. Yet these were contributing to her breakouts. And, while many foods that contain cinnamaldehyde, such as tomato and citrus, are healthy foods, Mary didn't realise that the natural food chemicals in them were also triggers for her rosacea.

NUTRITION

Mary was seeing a GP and a dermatologist, who was prescribing topical creams, but without nutritional support they weren't working as well as they could have. Mary didn't realise initially that she was coming to see me for help with her rosacea — her GP referred her to me for her weight gain, but her weight *did* seem to tie in with her skin. Mary was a sensible eater, focusing on high-fibre foods and keeping her dietary intake of saturated fats low; her cholesterol was low as a result. No one would have thought to look at her metabolic health, because she didn't look as if she had those issues. But it became apparent that she was starting to head in that direction.

Together with Mary's GP, I looked at underlying insulin resistance as the cause of her ongoing easy weight gain, hot flushes, midriff expansion and sugar cravings. Alongside the medical checks, a simple diet consisting of low-GI foods, balanced protein and good fats helped her to start regulating her weight, particularly around her waist. As a woman approaches menopause her body will often change from pear shape to apple shape — putting weight on around the middle instead of the hips, thighs and bust.

Research has found links between insulin and rosacea, and this helped Mary to make sense of what was happening to her. As a result we prescribed a balanced eating plan for her insulin resistance, and identified food triggers. This armed her with a way to manage the breakouts.

The other strategy we found effective was regular use of probiotics. Whenever Mary needed a course of antibiotics for her rosacea, we made sure she had a high-fibre diet and regular probiotics to manage her IBS. We found that when her tummy felt better, it showed in her skin.

RESULT

After around three months Mary was having fewer flare ups. We had been able to figure out her trigger foods, meaning she could still go out with her friends and enjoy wining and dining.

We were able to address her weight and her skin with one simple approach. Because we were reducing inflammation in her body, the osteoarthritis pain she was also experiencing eased, which, in turn, encouraged her to get back to regular exercise. All of this resulted in a bonus weight loss of 7 to 10 kilograms, and her waist measurement went down from 90cm to 80cm. She's been able to maintain her weight in the long term, to go on an overseas holiday and just enjoy life again.

HIDRADENITIS SUPPURATIVA :
When is a boil not just a boil?

If you can pronounce this condition, you've officially graduated from integumentary class. Hidradenitis suppurativa may be uncommon — it affects just 1–4 per cent of the population globally — but that doesn't make it any less serious. This chronic inflammatory follicular disorder forms in a similar way to acne. When hair follicles get blocked, they can rupture and leak into the dermis, causing swelling, nodules and painful tunnelling wounds. Often the disease begins gradually, perhaps as boils that won't go away or recur in the same places. These lesions are very painful, generally forming under the armpits or in the groin region. It is also common for hidradenitis suppurativa to form on the breasts, around the nipples, on the buttocks, inner thighs and genital area. In more severe cases, abscesses that discharge foul-smelling pus can develop, which often leaves purple scarring and hyperpigmented skin behind. Understandably, hidradenitis suppurativa affects not only people's physical health, but has a serious impact on their psychological and emotional wellbeing too.

LIFESTYLE It is understood that hormones, in particular androgens (male hormones), are responsible for activating this terrible skin condition, along with inflammation and autoimmune problems. Interestingly, the same hormones associated with teenage acne can become an inflammatory disorder that develops in the hair follicles and manifest as boils. Other factors that can increase the risk of hidradenitis suppurativa are smoking, obesity and having a family history of the condition. The onset usually occurs in the early twenties, and it is more commonly seen in females.

MEDICATION Typically, doctors will prescribe antibiotic gels or lotions, or oral antibiotics. If the condition is more severe, steroid injections might be used on the lesions. Some abscesses may need to be manually drained, while lesions that are most progressed and showing no signs of improvement with medical therapy could require surgical procedures and laser therapy. Anti-inflammatory medications are effective at reducing the severity of lesions, but they appear to be only a temporary solution; people often report a recurrence in the condition once they discontinue the medications.

When androgens (such as testosterone) occur in excess in females, this contributes to conditions such as PCOS and acne.

Interestingly, and not surprisingly, this might be why it is common for many people with hidradenitis suppurativa to also have PCOS, acne, or other insulin- and immune-system-related skin problems, such as psoriasis. It is thought that refined carbohydrates can exacerbate hidradenitis suppurativa.

Beneficial measures include wearing loose-fitting cotton clothing, losing weight and stopping smoking. Exercise, resistance training in particular, is a key component of treatment — those with hidradenitis suppurativa have been found to have significantly lower muscle and bone mass than those without the condition. Moreover, exercise and any subsequent weight loss will have a positive effect on insulin resistance and PCOS, as we know they often go hand in hand.

NUTRITION As with PCOS and acne, eliminating foods that might be contributing to insulin spikes and inflammatory responses is a key treatment. This could mean removing processed carbohydrates and refined sugar. In addition, yeast has been found to be a contributing factor. One study followed 12 patients after surgery for lesions. All followed an elimination diet post-surgery, avoiding any foods containing brewer's yeast. The skin of all patients quickly stabilised and within one year they had complete regression of their lesions.

HIDRADENITIS SUPPURATIVA
LAURA

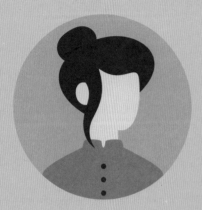

Laura was 25 years old, studying to be a nurse and working casually in a cafe. She was struggling with obesity, acne and low self-esteem. Compounding her low self-esteem, Laura had recurring boils in her groin region that appeared red, angry and inflamed. She was referred to me by her dermatologist because she had an autoimmune history of polycystic ovaries and insulin resistance.

SYMPTOMS AND TRIGGERS

Laura was pretty upset by the time she met me — not only was she troubled by her weight, but she now had these boils and felt she couldn't wear nice clothes or show her skin. It took a long time to get the diagnosis, because when is a boil just a boil, and when is it an ongoing condition? It's a challenge, managed by both a GP and a dermatologist for the hormonal (insulin) and autoimmune components. She was finding it frustrating to be controlled by this skin condition that required such regular testing and treatment. Laura had already been through many

frustrating dieting experiences since she was young; she often felt 'unclean' and had tried different ways to cleanse herself, ending up in a vicious cycle of binge eating and self-loathing.

Laura's health issue was overwhelming her; her skin condition was driven by her hormones, her immune system and also her nutrition. My role was to get Laura into a healthy pattern of eating, encourage her to take the medication to deal with her insulin resistance and to have injections from the dermatologist, as well as to follow up on further endocrine investigations.

TREATMENT

Weight loss was important for Laura. We looked at providing low-GI carbohydrates, balanced lean protein and a good-fat eating plan. The binge eating also needed to be addressed by a specialist eating-disorder psychologist.

Getting Laura to exercise was also challenging, when she didn't want to get sweaty and feel unclean. The psychologist helped her along the way, worked to keep her motivated and to get into a better pattern of eating by involving her family to help her. Her mother and father had both been diagnosed with diabetes and her sister had PCOS issues; so we were able to get the whole group behind her.

RESULT

Laura learned to trust food again and feel full and happy without bingeing and seeing food as the enemy. Once her condition went into remission, she found she could keep going with her food plan and it even got easier along the way. She eventually felt confident enough to get into her swimmers and go to the beach with her friends.

Dos and don'ts for your skin condition

CONDITION	FOODS TO AVOID	FOODS THAT MAY HELP	NUTRITIONAL SUPPORTS
Psoriasis	• Gluten (if you test positive for serologic markers of gluten sensitivity) • Alcohol • Nightshade plants (eggplant, tomato) • Processed sugar	• Mediterranean diet (high in extra virgin olive oil, fresh vegetables, legumes, seafood, nuts) • Low-GI carbohydrates	• Vitamin D (if deficient) • Indigo naturalis • Meditation • Acupuncture • Metformin • Omega-3 • Curcumin
Acne	• High-GI carbohydrates	• Adequate protein • Low-GI carbohydrates	• Zinc
Polycystic ovary syndrome (PCOS)	• High-GI carbohydrates • Trans fats • Saturated fatty acids	• Foods containing omega-3 polyunsaturated fatty acids • Low-GI carbohydrates and wholegrains	• Metformin • *Vitex agnus-castus*
Dermatitis herpetiformis	• Gluten	• Gluten-free diet	
Eczema	• Milk, eggs, wheat, soy, seafood, nuts • Food chemicals	• Probiotics and prebiotics • Low-GI carbohydrates	• Vitamin D • Keep a food-trigger journal to help identify intolerances • Avoid fragrance in washing powders

CONDITION	FOODS TO AVOID	FOODS THAT MAY HELP	NUTRITIONAL SUPPORTS
Hives	**ACUTE** • **In adults:** shellfish, freshwater fish, berries, nuts, peanuts, pork, chocolate, tomatoes, spices, food additives, alcohol • **In children:** milk, eggs, wheat, soy, seafood, nuts **CHRONIC** • Foods with salicylate, amine and glutamate	• Probiotics and prebiotics • Low-GI carbohydrates • Gluten-free diet	• Keep a food-trigger journal to help identify and avoid food intolerances
Rosacea	• Hot beverages • Alcohol • Spices and spicy foods, sauces • Foods containing capsaicin (capsicum/ peppers, chillies, paprika) • Foods containing cinnamaldehyde (cinnamon, citrus, tomatoes, chocolate)	• Low-GI carbohydrates • High-fibre foods	• Antibiotics (if there are gut issues such as *Helicobacter pylori*, or SIBO is present) • Omega-3: fish oil and flaxseed oil • Zinc • Probiotics and prebiotics • Metformin
Hidradenitis suppurativa	• Processed sugar • Foods containing yeast	• Low-GI carbohydrates	• Zinc

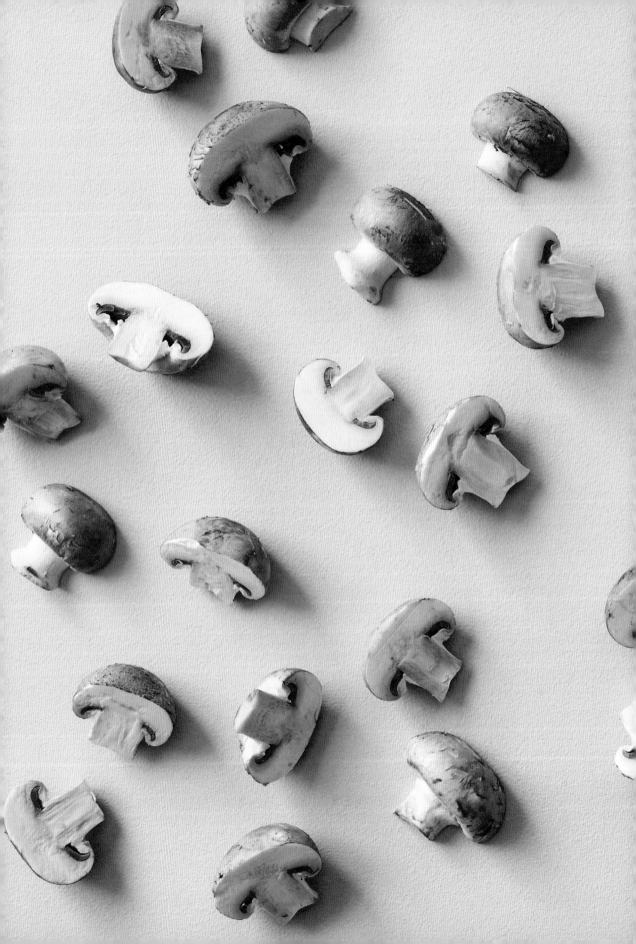

MEAL PLANS

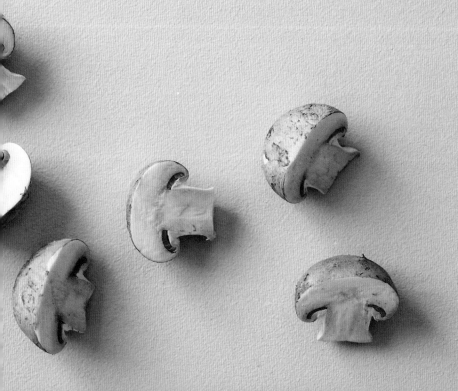

WEEK 1:
Getting started with happy tummies and healthy skin

	MONDAY	TUESDAY	WEDNESDAY
Breakfast	Apple Pie Smoothie (page 105) + 1 slice wholegrain bread with Vegemite + ¼ cup cottage cheese	Breakfast Toastie (page 126) + 1 glass low-fat milk	Apple & Almond Bircher Muesli (page 101) + ½ cup low-fat milk
Morning tea	3–4 wholegrain crispbreads with ¼ cup hummus + 100g lean leg ham + tomato slices	1 piece fruit + 1 small handful almonds	½ cup hummus with pitta crisps and veggie sticks
Lunch	The Reuben on Rye (page 180)	Lamb Wraps with Tzatziki Sauce (page 172)	Stuffed Mushrooms (page 155) (pictured)
Afternoon tea	Banana Nut Protein Pancakes (page 117)	1 small tub low-fat yoghurt	1 slice wholegrain bread + half a banana + ¼ cup cottage cheese
Dinner	Lamb Skewers with Pomegranate Tabbouleh (page 191)	Grilled Salmon with Apple Slaw (page 199) (pictured)	Dukkah Roast Chicken with Root Vegetable Crumble (page 200)
Supper	Kiwifruit, Strawberry and Basil Pops (page 227) (pictured)	4 wholegrain crackers + 2 tablespoons hummus	1 slice wholegrain toast + 1 tablespoon peanut butter

Deciding what to cook can sometimes be more taxing than the actual cooking. When you are tired or busy, it can be hard to plan ahead. The following 4 weeks of meal plans aim to take the decision-making out of your day and help you get started on the road to healthy skin using the simple recipes that follow. These plans are based on the average daily energy requirements for an adult of 8000 kilojoules (2000 calories) . Depending on your personal exercise habits and nutrition requirements, you might need to eat less or more. An Accredited Practising Dietitian can help you tailor these guidelines to your needs.

THURSDAY	FRIDAY	SATURDAY	SUNDAY
Spinach, Mushroom & Ricotta Omelette on Rye (page 121)	Latte Revitaliser (page 109) + 1 slice wholegrain raisin toast + 1 tablespoon low-fat cream cheese	Za'atar-rolled Eggs with Beetroot and Barley (page 130)	Blueberry & Pomegranate Smoothie Bowl (page 110) (pictured)
Fruit Dip (page 138)	Ham, Cheese & Tomato Mini Breakfast Quiches (page 133) (pictured)	Raspberry, Watermelon & Mint Smoothie (page 102)	Smoked Salmon Cream Cheese Bagel (page 114)
Leftover Roast Chicken Dinner Toastie (page 175)	Thai Beef Noodle Salad (page 147)	Vegetarian Buddha Bowl (page 167)	Curried Chicken & Mango Salad (page 140)
1 cup roasted chickpeas + ¼ cup grated low-fat cheddar cheese	1 piece fruit + 1 small handful nuts	Smashed Pumpkin with Feta & Pepita Dukkah (page 168) (pictured)	1 cup grapes + 1 slice low-fat cheese
Steak with Salsa Verde & White Beans (page 195) (pictured)	Tofu & Eggplant Curry with Zoodles (page 187)	Crispy Fish Tacos (page 196)	Corned Beef with Roasted Brussels Sprouts (page 192)
Cacao Banana Smoothie Bowl (page 97)	Roasted Grapes with Ricotta & French Toast (page 223)	2 Fig & Brazil Nut Bombs (page 224)	Parfait Your Way (page 139)

WEEK 2:

Challenging sugar cravings and enjoying low-GI carbs

	MONDAY	TUESDAY	WEDNESDAY
Breakfast	Raspberry, Watermelon & Mint Smoothie (page 102) + 1 slice wholegrain bread with Vegemite + ¼ cup cottage cheese	Banana Nut Protein Pancakes (page 117) *(pictured)*	Overnight Peaches & Cream Oats (page 98)
Morning tea	200g low-fat yoghurt + 1 serve fresh fruit	Sliced apple + 1 tablespoon almond butter	1 serve fresh fruit + 1 small handful almonds
Lunch	Vietnamese Chicken Salad Pitta (page 148)	Leftover Korean Beef Bibimbap (page 188)	Leftover White Bean Soup with Kale Pesto (page 216) *(pictured)*
Afternoon tea	Wholegrain nut snack bar + 1 serve fresh fruit	200g low-fat yoghurt + 1 serve fresh fruit	2 wholegrain crackers with ricotta + ½ sliced banana
Dinner	Korean Beef Bibimbap (page 188) *(pictured)*	White Bean Soup with Kale Pesto (page 216)	Mediterranean Chicken Pizza (page 211)
Supper	1 piece wholegrain raisin toast + 1 teaspoon butter + 1 slice low-fat cheese	Parfait Your Way (page 139)	2 cups popcorn with 1 teaspoon olive oil

THURSDAY	FRIDAY	SATURDAY	SUNDAY
2 slices wholegrain toast + ¼ avocado, smashed	1 cup wholegrain cereal + 1 cup high-protein milk + fresh berries	Sweet Potato Haloumi Hash with Fried Eggs (page 125)	Vegetarian Breakfast Burrito Bowl (page 122) *(pictured)*
½ cup low-fat hummus + pitta crisps + veggie sticks	200g low-fat yoghurt + 1 serve fresh fruit	1 serve fresh fruit + small handful almonds	1 slice wholegrain toast + peanut butter
Leftover Mediterranean Chicken Pizza (page 211)	Turkey, Cranberry, Cream Cheese & Alfalfa Sandwich (page 179)	Summer Pea, Mint & Goat's Cheese Tartine (page 171) *(pictured)*	Chicken Teriyaki Poke Bowl (page 164)
Wholegrain nut snack bar + 1 serve fresh fruit	1 slice reduced-fat cheese + 2 wholegrain crackers + fresh berries	Fruit Dip (page 138)	200g low-fat yoghurt + 1 serve fresh fruit
Lamb Fattoush (page 150) *(pictured)*	Crumbed Fish with Sweet Potato Chips (page 208) *(pictured)*	Stuffed Mushrooms (page 154)	Salmon, Dill & Zucchini Frittata (page 159)
Raw Carrot Cake with Lemon Ricotta Frosting (page 219)	1 cup Roasted Chickpeas (page 136)	Raw Carrot Cake with Lemon Ricotta Frosting (page 219)	Cacao Banana Smoothie Bowl (page 97)

WEEK 3:
Fibre, prebiotics and probiotics for gut health

	MONDAY	TUESDAY	WEDNESDAY
Breakfast	Apple & Almond Bircher Muesli (page 101)	2 slices wholegrain bread + 2 slices reduced-fat cheese + tomato	Vegetarian Breakfast Burrito Bowl (page 122)
Morning tea	2 wholegrain crackers + ¼ avocado + tomato slices	1 serve fresh fruit + 100g low-fat Greek yoghurt	2 slices wholegrain raisin toast + reduced-fat cream cheese
Lunch	Moroccan Chickpea Salad (page 144)	The Reuben on Rye (page 180)	Roast Beef Roll with Beetroot (page 176) *(pictured)*
Afternoon tea	200g low-fat yoghurt + 1 serve fresh fruit	2 wholegrain crackers + ¼ avocado + tomato	Wholegrain nut snack bar + 1 serve fresh fruit
Dinner	Cheeky Chow Mein (page 204) *(pictured)*	Black Bean Chilli with Cauliflower Rice (page 183)	Dukkah Roast Chicken with Root Vegetable Crumble (page 200)
Supper	1 cup Sweet Potato Chips (page 136)	Choc Banana Soft-serve (page 220) *(pictured)*	2 scoops low-fat vanilla ice cream + 1 cup berries

THURSDAY	FRIDAY	SATURDAY	SUNDAY
½ cup fruit-free muesli + 200g low-fat, high-protein yoghurt + 1 cup fruit salad	Apple Pie Smoothie (page 105) + 1 slice wholegrain bread with Vegemite + ¼ cup cottage cheese	Za'atar-rolled Eggs with Beetroot & Barley (page 130)	Smoked Salmon & Caper Omelette (page 118)
2 cups popcorn with 1 teaspoon olive oil	Wholegrain nut snack bar + 1 serve fresh fruit	200g low-fat yoghurt + 1 serve fresh fruit	Apple slices + 1 tablespoon almond butter
Quinoa, Broccoli and Haloumi Salad (page 152) (pictured)	Warm Salmon & Potato Salad with Sauerkraut (page 156)	Tuna Poke Bowl (page 160)	Turkey, Cranberry, Cream Cheese & Alfalfa Sandwich (page 179)
Pear slices + 1 tablespoon reduced-fat cream cheese + 1 tablespoon walnuts	200g low-fat yoghurt + 1 serve fresh fruit	¼ cup trail mix + 100g low-fat yoghurt	2 wholegrain crackers + ricotta + ½ sliced banana
Make-at-home Pad Thai (page 203)	Salmon, Dill & Zucchini Frittata (page 159) (pictured)	Steak with Salsa Verde and White Beans (page 195)	Pork Chops with Braised Cabbage & Apples (page 207) (pictured)
Banoffee Pots (page 106)	1 glass reduced-fat milk + 1–2 wholegrain crispbreads	Raw Carrot Cake with Lemon Ricotta Frosting (page 219) (pictured)	Cacao Banana Smoothie Bowl (page 97)

WEEK 4 :
Concentrating on healthy fats

	MONDAY	TUESDAY	WEDNESDAY
Breakfast	Apple & Almond Bircher Muesli (page 101) (*pictured*)	Latte Revitaliser (page 109) + 1 slice wholegrain raisin toast	Spinach, Mushroom & Ricotta Omelette on Rye (page 121)
Morning tea	Wholegrain nut snack bar + 1 serve fresh fruit	2 cups Kale Chips (page 137)	200g low-fat yoghurt + 1 serve fresh fruit
Lunch	Tuna Niçoise Salad (page 143)	Leftover Lentil Shepherd's Pie (page 185)	Smoked Salmon Cream Cheese Bagel (page 114)
Afternoon tea	Smashed Pumpkin with Feta and Pepita Dukkah (page 168)	Fruit Dip (page 138)	¼ cup trail mix
Dinner	Lentil Shepherd's Pie with Cheesy Cauliflower Crust (page 185)	Crispy Fish Tacos (page 196) (*pictured*)	Lamb Skewers with Pomegranate Tabbouleh (page 191) (*pictured*)
Supper	2 scoops low-fat vanilla ice cream + 1 cup berries	1 cup Sweet Potato Chips (page 136)	Parfait Your Way (page 139)

THURSDAY	FRIDAY	SATURDAY	SUNDAY
¼ avocado, smashed + 2 pieces sourdough toast	Dippy Eggs with Crunchy Seed Soldiers (page 113)	Ham, Cheese & Tomato Mini Breakfast Quiches (page 133)	Ricotta, Eggplant & Olive Bruschetta with Eggs (page 129) (pictured)
2 Ham, Cheese & Tomato Mini Breakfast Quiches (page 133)	Raspberry, Watermelon & Mint Smoothie (page 102) (pictured)	200g low-fat yoghurt + 1 serve fresh fruit	Pear slices + reduced-fat cream cheese + 1 tablespoon walnuts
Salmon Poke Bowl (page 163) (pictured)	Smashed Pumpkin with Feta and Pepita Dukkah (page 168)	Leftover Pasta with Chicken, Roast Peppers & Goat's Cheese (page 212)	Leftover Thai Beef Noodle Salad (page 147)
Apple slices + 1 tablespoon almond butter	1 piece wholegrain raisin toast + 1 teaspoon butter + 1 slice reduced-fat cheese	½ pitta bread + 1 banana + ¼ cup cottage cheese	1 cup milk + ¼ cup trail mix
Fool's Pho (page 215)	Pasta with Chicken, Roast Peppers & Goat's Cheese (page 212)	Thai Beef Noodle Salad (page 147)	Grilled Salmon with Apple Slaw & Pickled Onions (page 199)
Roasted Grapes with Ricotta & French Toast (page 223)	Parfait Your Way (page 139)	1 glass reduced-fat milk + Fig & Brazil Nut Bombs (page 224) (pictured)	Cacao Banana Smoothie Bowl (page 97)

Weekly shopping list
put your pantry and fridge to work

Fruit	Legumes	Vegetables
Apples	Black beans	Beetroot
Bananas	Cannellini beans	Broccoli
Fresh or frozen berries	Chickpeas	Carrot
Dates	Edamame	Cauliflower
Grapes	Kidney beans	Cucumber
Lemons	Lentils	Eggplant (aubergine)
Limes	Soy beans	Garlic
Mango		Ginger
Peaches		Green beans
Pears		Herbs
Pomegranate		Kale
Watermelon		Cos lettuce
		Mushrooms
		Onion
		Peas
		Pumpkin (squash)
		Rocket (arugula)
		Baby spinach
		Tomato
		Zucchini (courgette)

Spices & powders	Condiments	Fermented foods
Cacao nibs	Fish sauce	Kefir
Cacao powder	Pickled ginger	Kimchi
Cumin	Honey	Kombucha
Garam masala	Horseradish	Sauerkraut – red and white
Garlic	Maple syrup	
Paprika	Pomegranate molasses	
Thyme	Dijon mustard	
Turmeric	Seeded mustard	
	Soy sauce (salt-reduced)	
	White and red wine vinegar	

Low-GI carbohydrates	Non-wheat gluten-free carbohydrates	Vegetable carbohydrates
Barley	Egg noodles	Corn
Rye bread	Rice noodles	Potato
Sourdough bread	Soba noodles	Sweet potato
Soy linseed bread	Quinoa	
Wholegrain bread	Quinoa flakes	
Wholemeal bread	Puffed rice	
Wholegrain crispbreads	Basmati rice	
Natural muesli	Doongara (low-GI) rice	
Wholemeal pasta	Brown rice	
Wholemeal pitta bread		
Rolled oats		

Lean proteins	Dairy*	Good fats
Lean beef and mince	Cheddar cheese	Avocado
Chicken breast	Cottage cheese	Dukkah
Fish	Feta cheese	Nuts: almonds, Brazil nuts, walnuts
Lamb fillet	Ricotta cheese	
Pork chops	Kefir	Canola oil
Salmon	Milk	Extra virgin olive oil
Eggs	Greek yoghurt	Olive oil
Tofu	Natural yoghurt	Salmon
Vanilla protein powder		Seeds: chia, linseeds/flaxseeds, pepitas, sunflower
	* Choose low-fat options	Tahini

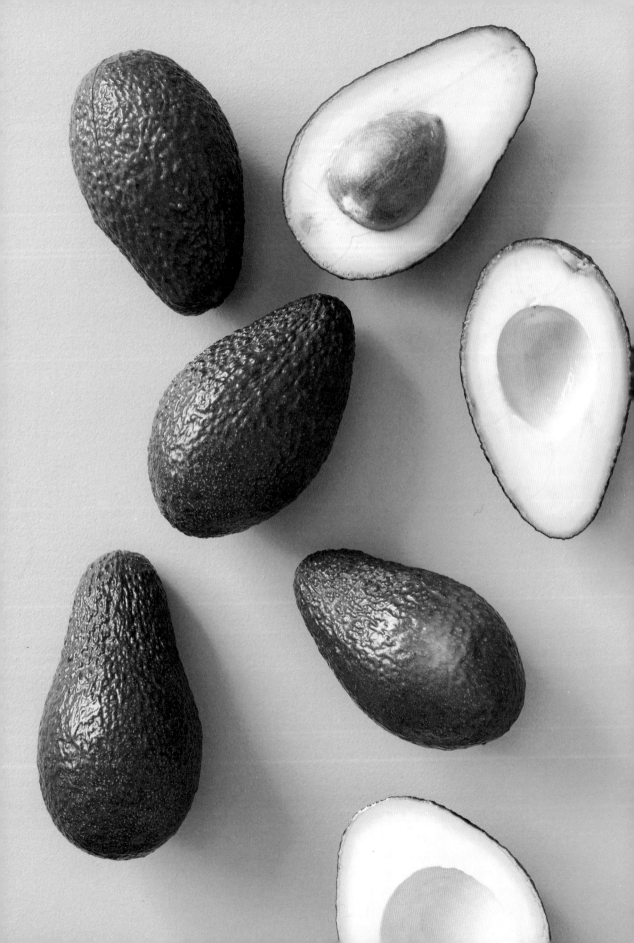

RECIPES

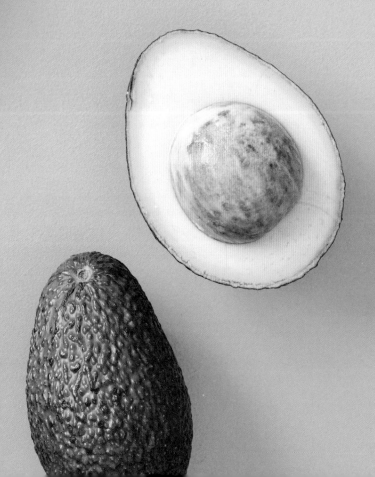

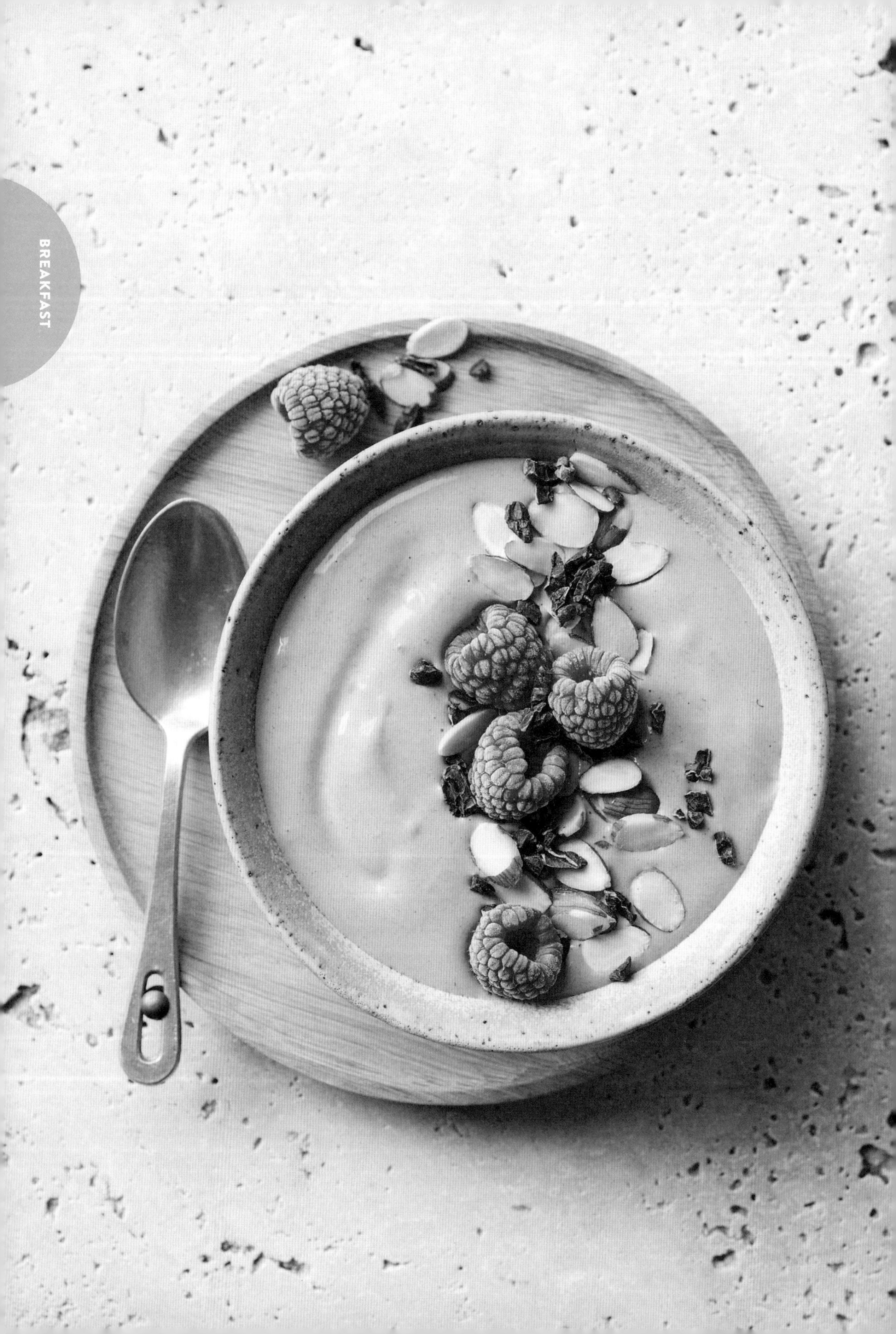

Cacao banana smoothie bowl : GF

Everybody is loving smoothie bowls right now, because they're downright delicious. But beware: they might seem healthy but commercial smoothie bowls can contain up to 120 grams of sugar. Spiking your blood glucose levels can lead to high insulin levels, leading to a cascade of hormonal changes that can trigger acne. This quick and easy recipe balances carbohydrate with protein, which can help prevent inflammation.

SERVES 2 PREP TIME: 5 MINS

1 frozen banana
1 tablespoon cacao powder
1 cup (260 g) low-fat Greek yoghurt
½ cup (50 g) vanilla protein powder
30 g (1 oz) cacao nibs
1 tablespoon flaked almonds
½ cup (125 g) frozen raspberries

Put the banana, cacao powder, yoghurt and protein powder into a blender and blend until smooth.

Pour into two bowls and scatter the cacao nibs, flaked almonds and frozen raspberries across the top.

ANALYSIS SUMMARY

(PER SERVE) ENERGY 1325 KJ (317 CAL), PROTEIN 21 G, TOTAL FAT 12 G, SATURATED FAT 5 G, CARBOHYDRATE 28 G, SUGARS 14 G, DIETARY FIBRE 5 G

Overnight peaches & cream oats

Looking to ramp up your oat consumption a notch? This recipe is everything you've ever wanted in a quick brekky. Creamy, fruity and crunchy, with every mouthful different from the one before, not only does it taste like Christmas, but it will keep your energy levels steady all day. This is super-easy to make the night before, saving you time in the morning. If you're gluten intolerant, use quinoa flakes instead of oats.

SERVES 2 PREP TIME: 5 MINS

¾ cup (75 g) rolled oats
1 cup (260 g) low-fat Greek yoghurt
1 peach, chopped
1 cup (250 ml) skim milk (or milk alternative)
½ cup (50 g) vanilla protein powder
pinch of nutmeg
1 tablespoon chia seeds
1 tablespoon flaxseeds (linseeds)

Put all the ingredients except the flaxseeds into a large bowl and mix well.

Spoon into jars, sprinkle with flaxseeds and refrigerate overnight before serving.

ANALYSIS SUMMARY

(PER SERVE) ENERGY 1633 KJ (390 CAL), PROTEIN 35 G, TOTAL FAT 8 G, SATURATED FAT 1 G, CARBOHYDRATE 39 G, SUGARS 17 G, DIETARY FIBRE 7 G

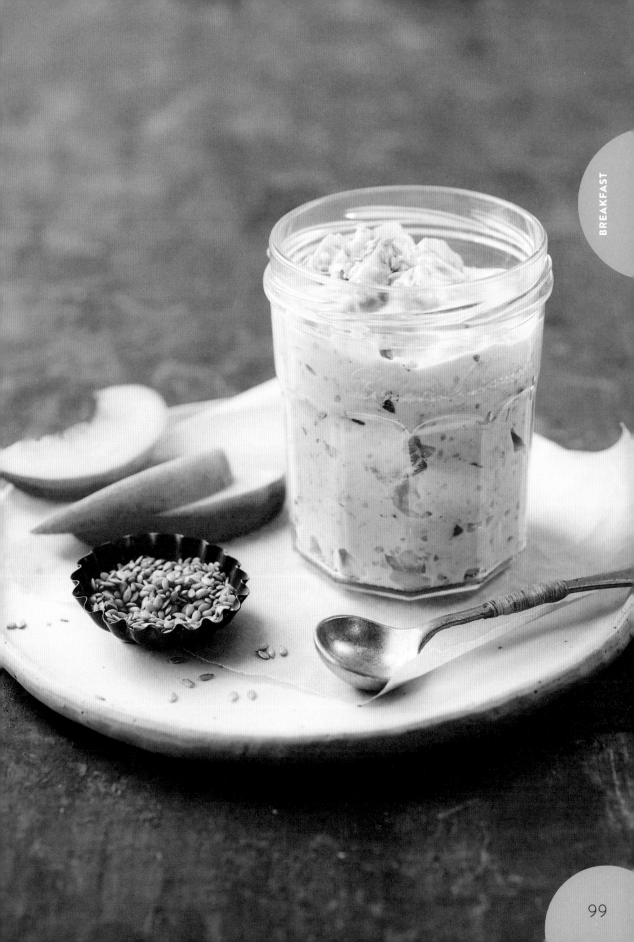

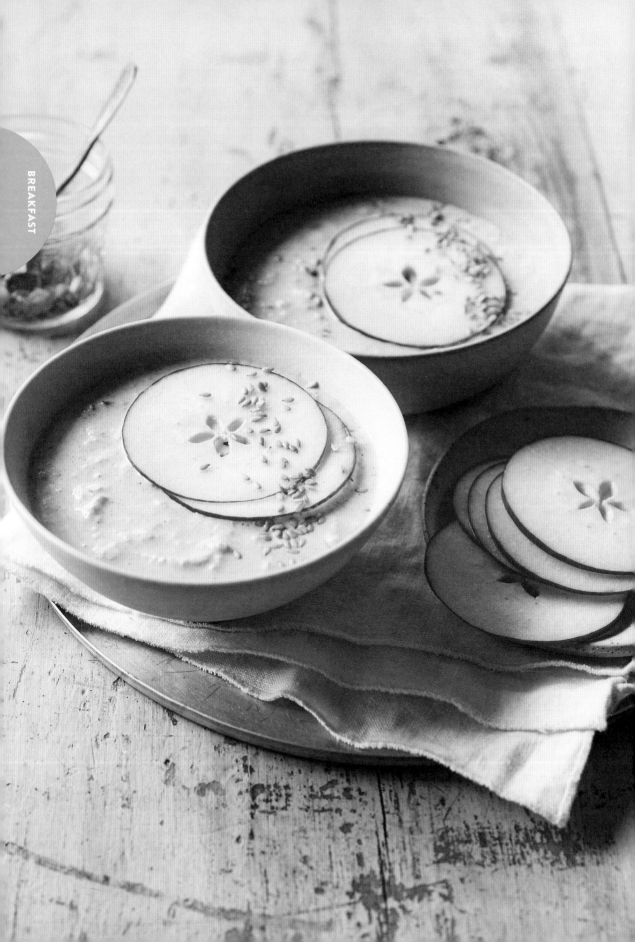

Apple & almond bircher muesli

Bircher muesli was created in the 1900s by a Swiss physician who claimed to have cured his own jaundice with apples. It is still renowned as a nourishing breakfast, packed full of vitamin C, fibre, protein and low-GI carbohydrates that are easily digested after overnight soaking. This recipe keeps it simple, original and delicious. If you're gluten intolerant, use quinoa flakes instead of oats.

SERVES 2 PREP TIME: 5 MINS

1 cup (250 ml) skim milk (or milk alternative)
½ cup (50 g) vanilla protein powder
1 apple, grated
½ cup (50 g) rolled oats
1 cup (260 g) low-fat Greek yoghurt
1 teaspoon ground cinnamon
3 tablespoons flaxseeds (linseeds)
finely sliced apple, to serve

Combine the milk and protein powder. Put the grated apple, oats, yoghurt and cinnamon in a large bowl, add the milk mixture and mix well.

Spoon into bowls or jars and refrigerate overnight before serving with flaxseeds and sliced apple.

ANALYSIS SUMMARY

(PER SERVE) ENERGY 1538 KJ (368 CAL), PROTEIN 27 G, TOTAL FAT 11 G, SATURATED FAT 1 G, CARBOHYDRATE 35 G, SUGARS 19 G, DIETARY FIBRE 6 G

Raspberry, watermelon & mint smoothie : GF

Smoothies are a great way to pack in extra fruit and vegetables, which are full of fibre, minerals and antioxidants that are beneficial for the skin. Raspberries, in particular, are rich in vitamin C and potassium, essential for cell regeneration. It's important to combine the carbohydrates we eat with a source of protein, as this helps reduce the glycaemic index of the meal.

SERVES 2 PREP TIME: 5 MINS

2 cups (250 g) frozen raspberries
½ cup (50 g) vanilla protein powder
1 cup (150 g) diced watermelon
1 handful mint
ice

Put all the ingredients in a blender with a handful of ice and blend. Add water, if necessary, to reach the consistency you like.

Pour into two glasses and enjoy.

ANALYSIS SUMMARY

(PER SERVE) ENERGY 615 KJ (147 CAL), PROTEIN 14 G, TOTAL FAT 1 G, SATURATED FAT 0.25 G, CARBOHYDRATE 15 G, SUGARS 14 G, DIETARY FIBRE 8 G

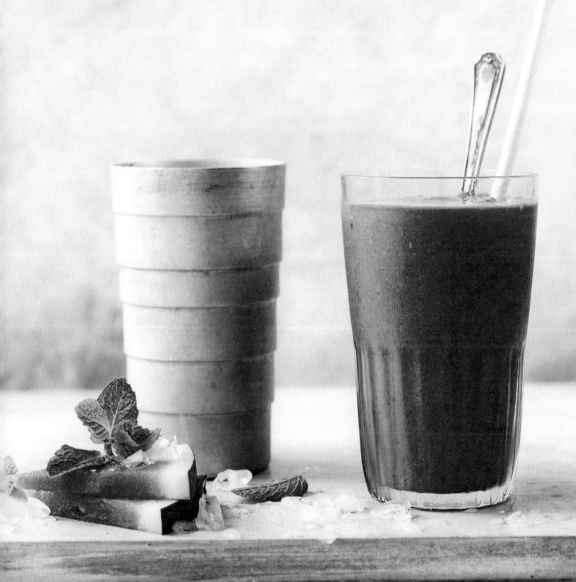

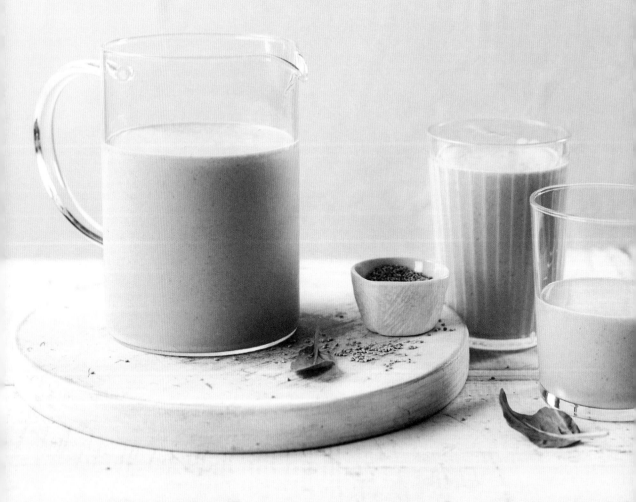

Apple pie smoothie : GF

This smoothie is great as a snack, or you can enjoy it alongside an omelette as a delicious balanced meal. It's high in vitamins A and C, which help fight oxidative stress in the skin. Vitamin C can also increase non-haem iron absorption, which helps to transport oxygen around the body and prevent iron deficiency.

SERVES 2 PREP TIME: 5 MINS

1 cup (45 g) baby spinach
1 green apple, core removed, chopped
1 cup (260 g) low-fat Greek yoghurt
4 tablespoons vanilla protein powder
pinch of nutmeg
1 tablespoon chia seeds
ice

Put all the ingredients in a blender with a handful of ice and blend. Add water, if necessary, to reach the consistency you like.

Pour into two glasses.

ANALYSIS SUMMARY

(PER SERVE) ENERGY 795 KJ (190 CAL), PROTEIN 19 G, TOTAL FAT 3 G, SATURATED FAT 1 G, CARBOHYDRATE 18 G, SUGARS 12 G, DIETARY FIBRE 6 G

Banoffee pots : GF

This smoothie is decadence in a glass – AND it's good for you! It's high in potassium, protein and calcium, which assist in the growth and repair of skin, as well as the production of sebum for skin hydration. Freezing bananas is a clever way to always have smoothie ingredients on hand. You can also use this recipe as a dessert option.

SERVES 2 PREP TIME: 5 MINS

1 frozen banana
½ cup (50 g) vanilla protein powder
2 cups (500 ml) skim milk (or milk alternative)
½ cup (130 g) low-fat Greek yoghurt
2 medjool dates, pitted
1 tablespoon chopped walnuts

Put all of the ingredients except the walnuts into a blender and mix until smooth. Add water, if necessary, to reach the consistency you like.

Pour into cups or glasses and scatter with chopped walnuts for crunch.

ANALYSIS SUMMARY

(PER SERVE) ENERGY 1098 KJ (262 CAL), PROTEIN 23 G, TOTAL FAT 5 G, SATURATED FAT 1 G, CARBOHYDRATE 30 G, SUGARS 25 G, DIETARY FIBRE 2 G

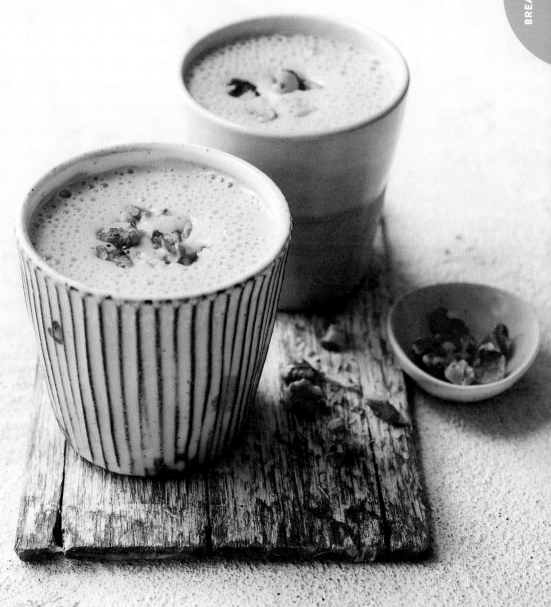

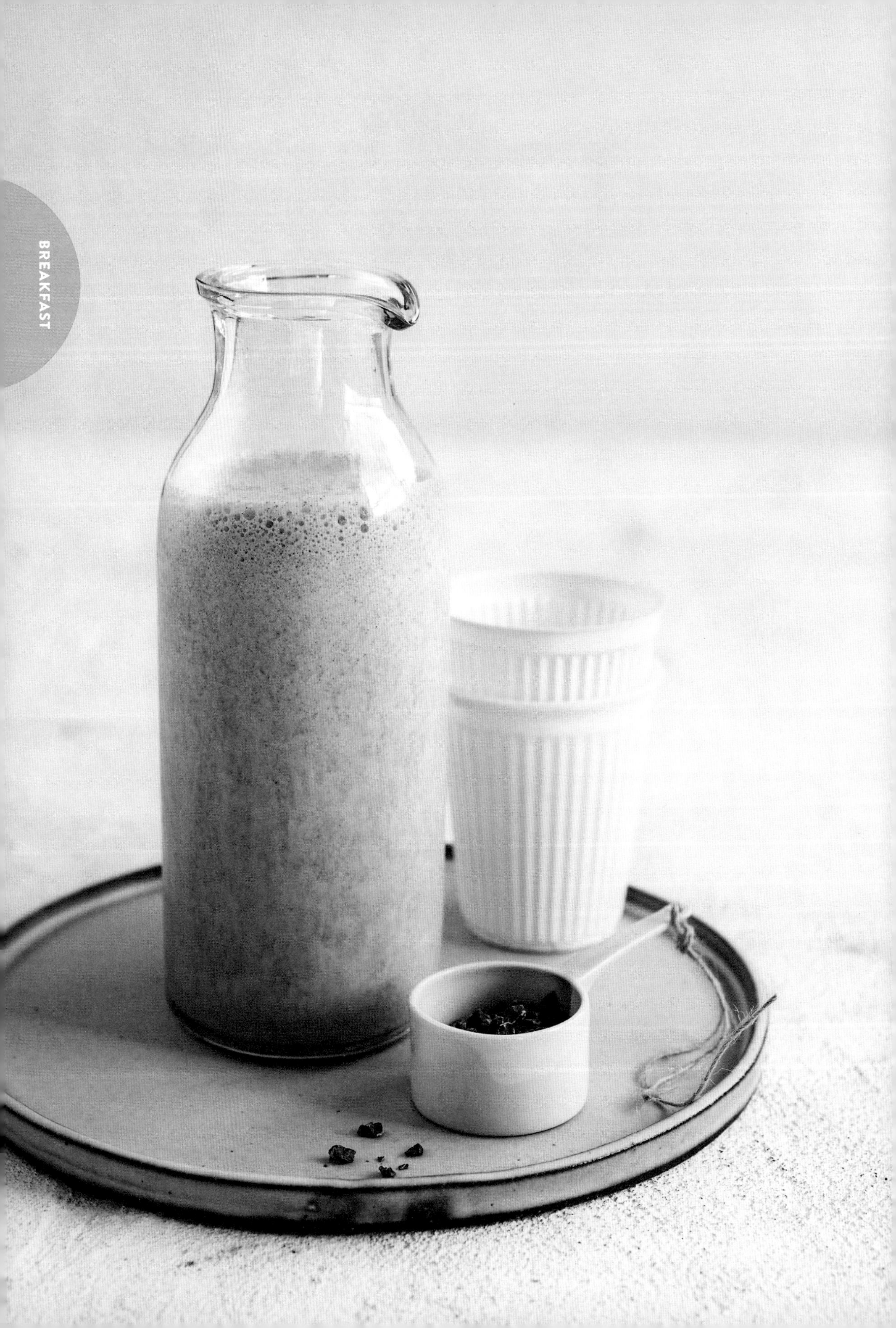

Latte revitaliser : GF

Both a sweet fix and an energy boost, this is a perfect pick-me-up breakfast or snack.
The ingredients are especially high in potassium, which is an electrolyte important for
muscle contraction and conducting messages around the body. The cacao nibs are also
rich in antioxidants, which are great for the skin.

SERVES 2 PREP TIME: 5 MINS

1 frozen banana
2 espresso shots (60 ml)
½ cup (50 g) vanilla protein powder
2 cups (500 ml) skim milk (or milk alternative)
20 g (¾ oz) cacao nibs

Put all of the ingredients except the cacao nibs into a blender
and blend until smooth. Add water, if necessary, to reach the
consistency you like.

Pour into a jar or glass and sprinkle with cacao nibs for crunch.

ANALYSIS SUMMARY
(PER SERVE) ENERGY 1128 KJ (270 CAL), PROTEIN 27 G, TOTAL FAT 5 G, SATURATED FAT 3 G,
CARBOHYDRATE 28 G, SUGARS 20 G, DIETARY FIBRE 2 G

Blueberry & pomegranate smoothie bowl : GF

BREAKFAST

Fresh pomegranates and blueberries are the ultimate antioxidant hits to the nasty free radicals that age us over time. Add the omega-3s from chia seeds, which reduce inflammation and nourish the skin from the inside, and this is a bowl of youth. It's also an excellent source of fibre, which promotes a great gut microbiome too.

SERVES 2 PREP TIME: 10 MINS

1 pomegranate
1 cup (125 g) frozen blueberries
1 cup (260 g) low-fat Greek yoghurt
½ cup (50 g) vanilla protein powder
1 tablespoon chia seeds
2 tablespoons shredded coconut

Halve the pomegranate, collecting the juice in a bowl.

Pour the juice into a blender and add the blueberries, yoghurt and protein powder. Blend until smooth.

Tap out the pomegranate seeds into a bowl.

Pour the smoothie into small bowls and scatter with the pomegranate seeds, chia seeds and shredded coconut.

ANALYSIS SUMMARY _____

(PER SERVE) ENERGY 1140 KJ (272 CAL), PROTEIN 20 G, TOTAL FAT 8 G, SATURATED FAT 5 G, CARBOHYDRATE 25 G, SUGARS 18 G, DIETARY FIBRE 9 G

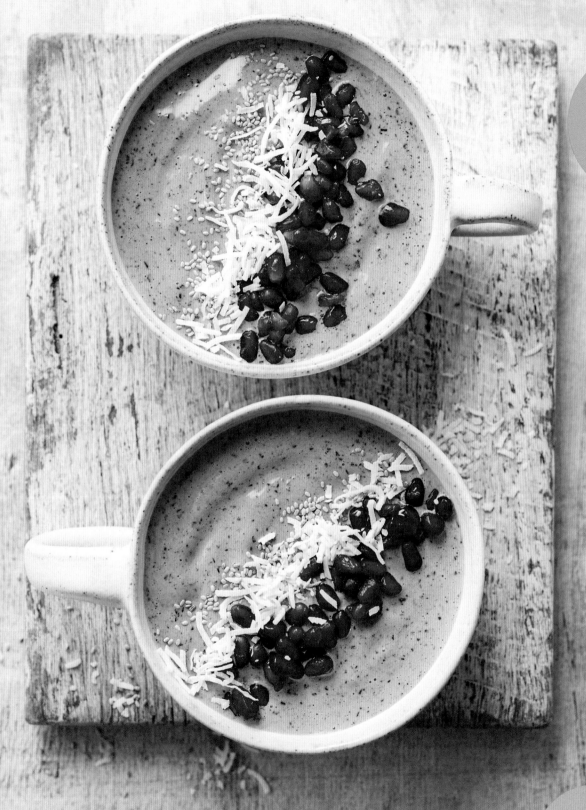

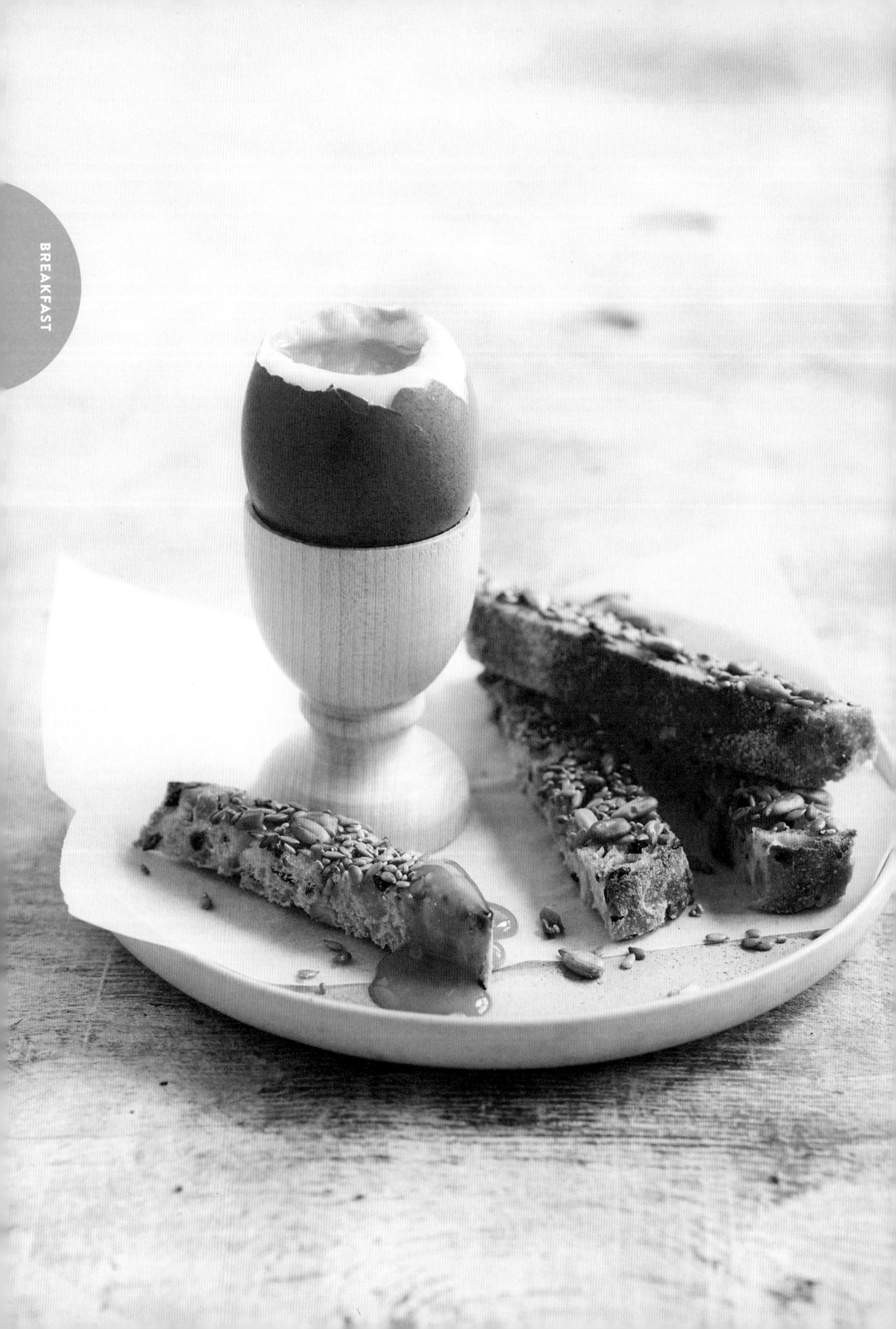

Dippy eggs with crunchy seed soldiers

This is a great brekky for supporting your gut microbiome and reducing inflammation. Low GI and rich in good fats, it's also an excellent way to boost your fibre intake for the day. Plus it's high in antioxidants for healthy skin.

SERVES 2 PREP TIME: 5 MINS COOKING TIME: 15 MINS

2 teaspoons olive oil spread
4 slices soy-linseed bread or gluten-free wholegrain bread
2 tablespoons mixed seeds (such as linseeds/flaxseeds, chia seeds and sunflower seeds)
4 large eggs

Preheat the grill to high.

Spread the olive oil spread over the bread and cut into fingers.

Spread the seeds into a shallow dish and coat the bread in seeds. Place on a baking tray and grill for 4–5 minutes, turning occasionally, until golden and crisp.

Meanwhile, put the eggs in a small saucepan, cover with cold water and place over high heat. When the water comes to the boil, take the pan off the heat and leave the eggs to sit in the water for 2 minutes.

Place the eggs in egg cups, cut off the tops and serve with the crunchy seed soldiers.

ANALYSIS SUMMARY

(PER SERVE) ENERGY 1312 KJ (314 CAL), PROTEIN 19 G, TOTAL FAT 15 G, SATURATED FAT 2 G, CARBOHYDRATE 23 G, SUGARS 2 G, DIETARY FIBRE 7 G

Smoked salmon cream cheese bagel

Go on, you know you want to! This recipe needs no introduction: the simple, delicious ingredients speak for themselves. I could tell you that it's low GI and high in omega-3, but who cares when it tastes this good?

SERVES 2 PREP TIME: 5 MINS COOKING TIME: 5 MINS

1 wholemeal or gluten-free bagel
2 tablespoons reduced-fat cream cheese
1 tomato, sliced
200 g (7 oz) smoked salmon
2 tablespoons chopped chives

Slice the bagel in half through the middle and toast both sides.

Spread with the cream cheese, then add the tomato slices and smoked salmon, and sprinkle with chives.

ANALYSIS SUMMARY ⎯⎯⎯⎯⎯⎯⎯⎯⎯⎯⎯⎯⎯⎯⎯⎯⎯⎯⎯⎯⎯⎯⎯⎯⎯

(PER SERVE) ENERGY 1648 KJ (392 CAL), PROTEIN 31 G, TOTAL FAT 15 G, SATURATED FAT 5 G, CARBOHYDRATE 32 G, SUGARS 5 G, DIETARY FIBRE 3 G

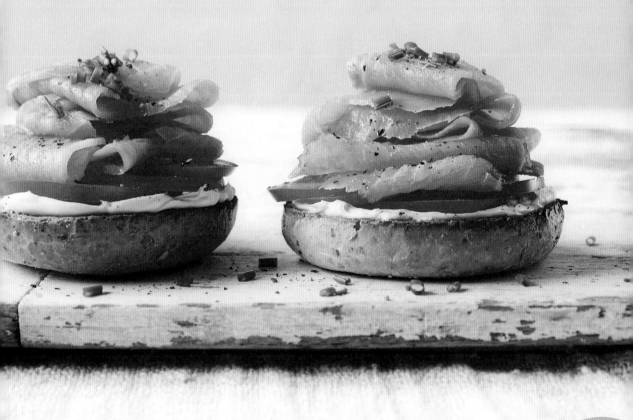

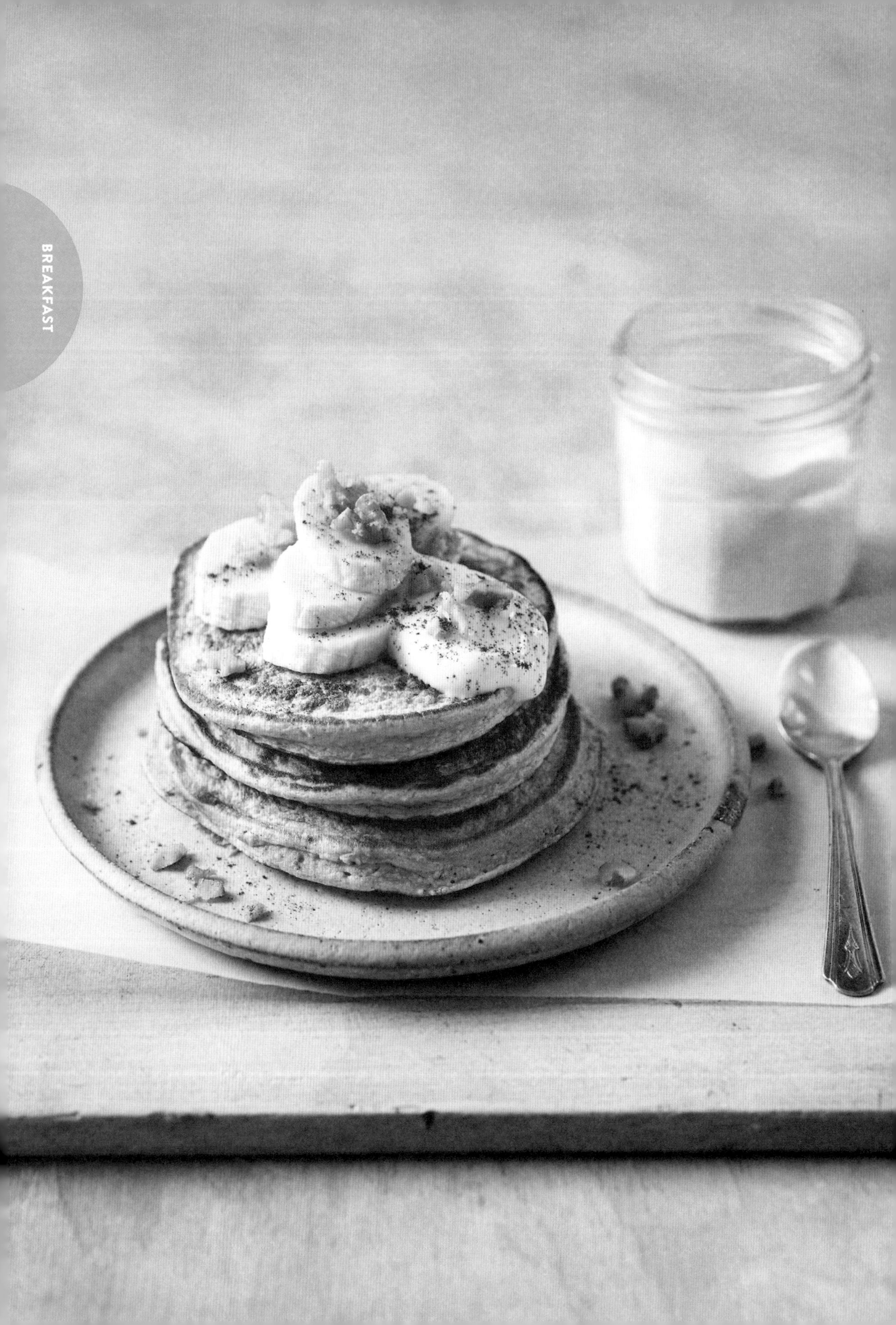

Banana nut protein pancakes

Yes, you can have your cake and eat it. The breakfast section wouldn't be complete without a pancake recipe and I think this one is a winner. A great alternative to flour, rolled oats are low GI and high in fibre, and they help to reduce bad cholesterol. Light, fluffy and comforting, these pancakes make a terrific nutritionally balanced breakfast. To make them gluten free, use quinoa flakes instead of oats. I use egg whites only for the extra protein boost, but you could use whole eggs.

SERVES 2 PREP TIME: **10 MINS** COOKING TIME: **15 MINS**

½ cup (50 g) rolled oats
6 large egg whites (or 4 large eggs)
3 tablespoons vanilla protein powder
2 small bananas
pinch of ground cinnamon
1 teaspoon vegetable oil
½ cup (130 g) low-fat Greek yoghurt
2 walnuts, chopped

Put the oats, egg whites, protein powder, 1 banana and the cinnamon in a blender and mix to a smooth batter.

Heat the oil in a non-stick frying pan over medium heat and pour ¼ cup batter into the pan. When large bubbles form on the surface of the pancake after about 3 minutes, flip the pancake over and cook until lightly golden on the other side. Cook the rest of the batter (depending on the size of your pan, you might be able to cook more than one at a time).

Slice the remaining banana. Serve the pancakes with sliced banana, yoghurt and walnuts.

ANALYSIS SUMMARY

(PER SERVE) ENERGY 1503 KJ (379 CAL), PROTEIN 28 G, TOTAL FAT 13 G, SATURATED FAT 1 G, CARBOHYDRATE 31 G, SUGARS 13 G, DIETARY FIBRE 5 G

Smoked salmon & caper omelette with roast potato gems : GF

This omelette is the ultimate meal for your skin. It combines protein for cell repair and growth, omega-3 for reduced inflammation, and healthy carbs for steady blood sugar levels. Don't be scared of potato: it's high in fibre, potassium and vitamin C, which all play a role in immunity and fluid regulation – so important when it comes to skin. I use egg white only, for the extra protein boost, but feel free to use whole eggs.

SERVES 2 PREP TIME: **10 MINS** COOKING TIME: **30 MINS**

2 large white potatoes, unpeeled, cut into cubes
2 teaspoons olive oil
6 large egg whites (or 4 large eggs)
150 g (5½ oz) smoked salmon
¼ red onion, finely sliced
2 tablespoons capers, rinsed
lemon wedges, to serve

Preheat the oven to 180°C (350°F) fan-forced and line a baking tray with baking paper.

Sprinkle the potato cubes with 1 teaspoon of oil and season with salt and pepper. Spread on the tray and bake for 25 minutes or until golden.

When the potatoes are cooked, heat the remaining oil in a large frying pan over medium heat. Whisk the egg whites with a pinch of salt.

Pour half the egg into the pan and swirl to coat the pan with a thin layer. Cook for 2 minutes or until the egg is just set, then lay half the salmon, onion and capers on top and allow to heat through. Fold the omelette in half and cook for a further 3 minutes or until the base is golden. Remove from the pan and keep warm while you make a second omelette.

Serve with roast potato gems and lemon wedges.

ANALYSIS SUMMARY _____

(PER SERVE) ENERGY 1610 KJ (383 CAL), PROTEIN 34 G, TOTAL FAT 13 G, SATURATED FAT 2 G, CARBOHYDRATE 31 G, SUGARS 4 G, DIETARY FIBRE 4 G

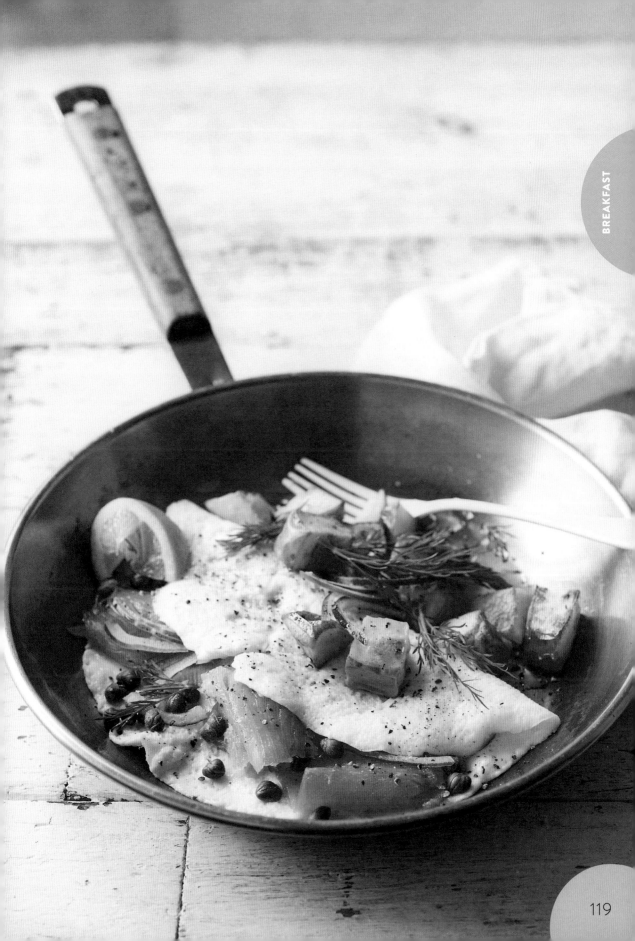

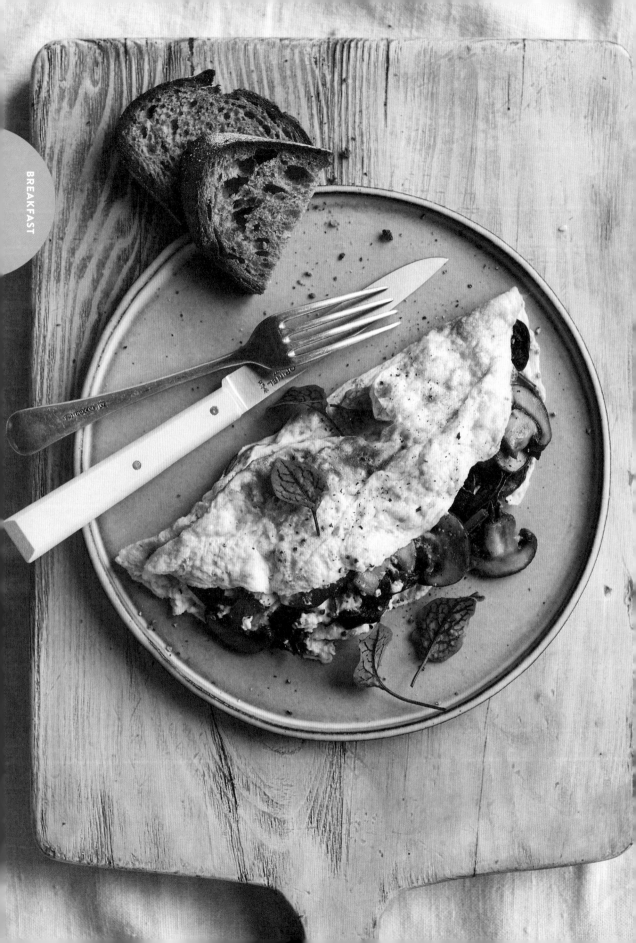

Spinach, mushroom & ricotta omelette on rye

Omelettes aren't just for weekend café brunches. Don't be intimidated: this recipe is so super-quick and easy you can make it on any day of the week. It's also packed full of protein, calcium, vegetables and low-GI carbs to keep you going through those midmorning munchies. I use egg white only, for the extra protein boost, but feel free to use whole eggs.

SERVES 2 PREP TIME: **5 MINS** COOKING TIME: **10 MINS**

1 garlic clove, crushed
1 cup (90 g) sliced mushrooms
1 cup (45 g) baby spinach
1 cup (230 g) reduced-fat ricotta cheese
6 large egg whites (or 4 large eggs)
2 teaspoons seeded mustard
1 teaspoon olive oil
2 thick slices rye bread or gluten-free
   wholegrain bread, toasted

Heat a large non-stick frying pan over medium heat and add the garlic, mushrooms and spinach. Cover with a lid and leave to steam for 3 minutes.

Tip the steamed vegetables into a bowl and mix with the ricotta.

In a separate bowl, whisk the egg whites with the mustard and a pinch of salt and pepper.

Return the pan to the heat and add the oil. Pour in half the egg, pushing it in from the sides until almost set.

Add half the vegetable mixture, then fold the omelette over the top and slide it onto a plate.

Repeat with the remaining mixture. Serve each omelette with a slice of toast.

ANALYSIS SUMMARY

(PER SERVE) ENERGY 1317 KJ (315 CAL), PROTEIN 26 G, TOTAL FAT 8 G, SATURATED FAT 3 G, CARBOHYDRATE 30 G, SUGARS 4 G, DIETARY FIBRE 5 G

Vegetarian breakfast
burrito bowl : GF

BREAKFAST

This recipe is a great combination of low-GI carbohydrates and lean protein, which assists in the slow release of glucose and regulates insulin response, helping you to feel full and happy. Legumes, such as black beans, are an excellent source of prebiotic fibre and fuel for your gut microbiome. This breakfast also makes a terrific last-minute pantry meal at any time of the day.

SERVES 2 PREP TIME: 5 MINS COOKING TIME: 5 MINS

125 g (4½ oz) tinned corn kernels, drained
125 g (4½ oz) tinned black beans, drained
1 tomato, chopped
½ red onion, finely chopped
1 small red chilli, seeded and chopped
1 lemon or lime, halved
200 g (7 oz) firm tofu
4 egg whites (or 2 large eggs)
2 teaspoons olive oil
¼ avocado, sliced or mashed

Mix together the corn, black beans, tomato, onion, chilli and the juice of 1 lemon or lime half.

In a separate bowl, mash the tofu with a fork and whisk in the egg whites. Season with salt and pepper.

Heat the oil in a non-stick frying pan over low to medium heat and add the tofu mixture to the pan, stirring constantly until the eggs have just set.

To serve, divide the corn and bean mixture between two bowls and place the scrambled tofu on top. Add a slice or dollop of avocado and serve with lemon or lime wedges.

ANALYSIS SUMMARY

(PER SERVE) ENERGY 1630 KJ (390 CAL), PROTEIN 29 G, TOTAL FAT 14 G, SATURATED FAT 2 G, CARBOHYDRATE 34 G, SUGARS 6 G, DIETARY FIBRE 15 G

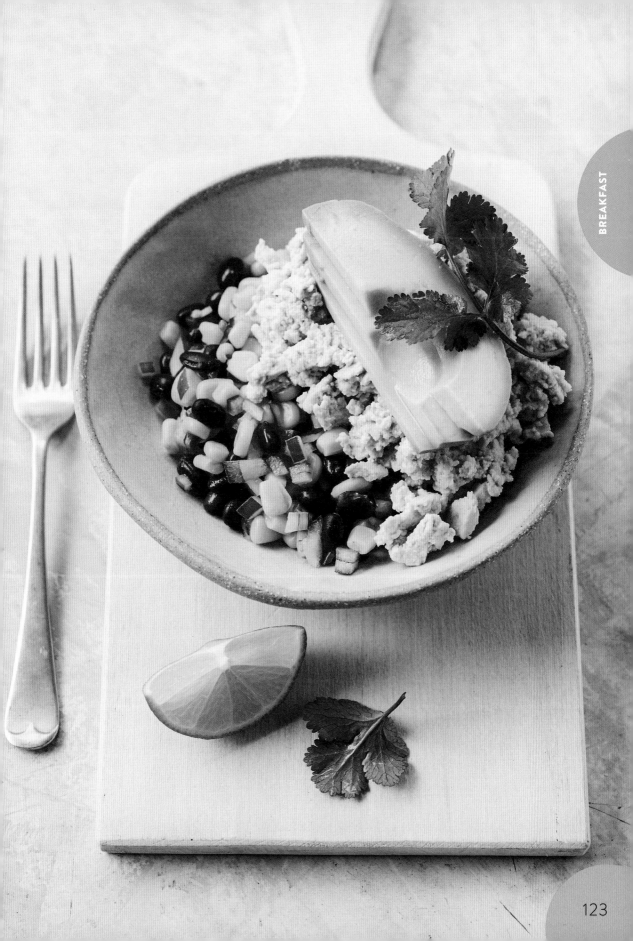

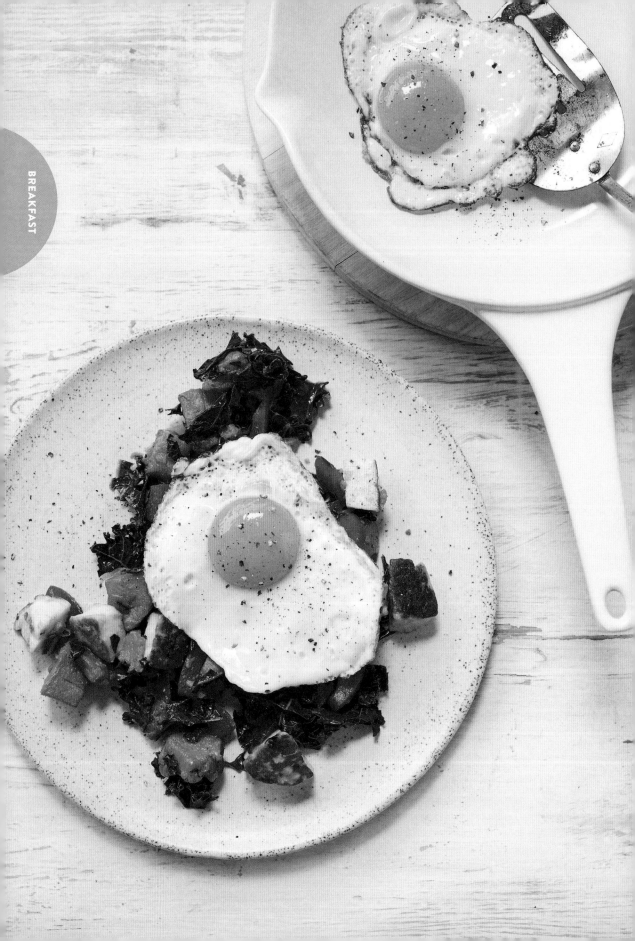

Sweet potato haloumi hash with fried eggs : GF

Ever wondered how to use up those leftover root veggies from the night before? This recipe is great for brekky and the hash can also be made in advance and reheated for busy days. Kale is a cruciferous 'protective' vegetable. It's high in prebiotics – essential for a healthy gut – as well as antioxidants such as vitamin C that protect our skin from free radicals. This meal is also rich in vitamin A, which can help with skin repair.

SERVES: **4** PREP TIME: **10 MINS** COOKING TIME: **15 MINS**

2 teaspoons olive oil
1 leftover large roast sweet potato, diced
100 g (3½ oz) haloumi cheese, diced
½ bunch kale, stalks removed and leaves chopped
1 large red capsicum (pepper), seeded and chopped
1 large spring onion (scallion), chopped
1 garlic clove, crushed
2 tablespoons balsamic vinegar
8 eggs

Heat 1 teaspoon of oil in a large frying pan over medium–high heat. Add the sweet potato and haloumi and sauté for 5–7 minutes until the sweet potato is heated through and the haloumi is beginning to brown.

Add the kale, capsicum, spring onion and garlic. Sauté for about 5 minutes until the kale has wilted. Add the balsamic vinegar and toss.

Spoon onto plates and keep warm while you fry the eggs.

Wipe out the pan and add the remaining 1 teaspoon oil. Fry the eggs for 2½ minutes until the whites are just set and yolks are still runny.

Top each serve of hash with two fried eggs.

ANALYSIS SUMMARY

(PER SERVE) ENERGY 1042 KJ (248 CAL), PROTEIN 19 G, TOTAL FAT 7 G, SATURATED FAT 3 G, CARBOHYDRATE 23 G, SUGARS 13 G, DIETARY FIBRE 9 G

Breakfast toastie

Let's face it, in the cooler months, there's nothing better than the smell of bread and cheese dancing together in toastie heaven. It can be tempting to grab one from a café on the way to work, but those are often high in saturated fat. Crunchy on the outside, warm and chewy on the inside, this healthy toastie is so easy to put together, there really is no excuse for not making your own. Look for a good-quality, low-sugar variety of tomato relish.

SERVES 2 PREP TIME: 5 MINS COOKING TIME: 5 MINS

1 tablespoon tomato relish
4 slices wholegrain bread or wholegrain gluten-free bread
40 g reduced-fat cheddar cheese, sliced
200 g (7 oz) leg ham
1 cup (35 g) rocket (arugula)

Spread the tomato relish over 2 slices of bread. Layer the cheese, ham and rocket on top and place the other 2 slices of bread on top.

Toast in a sandwich press for about 5 minutes or until the bread is golden and the cheese is melted.

ANALYSIS SUMMARY

(PER SERVE) ENERGY 1594 KJ (381 CAL), PROTEIN 32 G, TOTAL FAT 11 G, SATURATED FAT 5 G, CARBOHYDRATE 31 G, SUGARS 5 G, DIETARY FIBRE 7 G

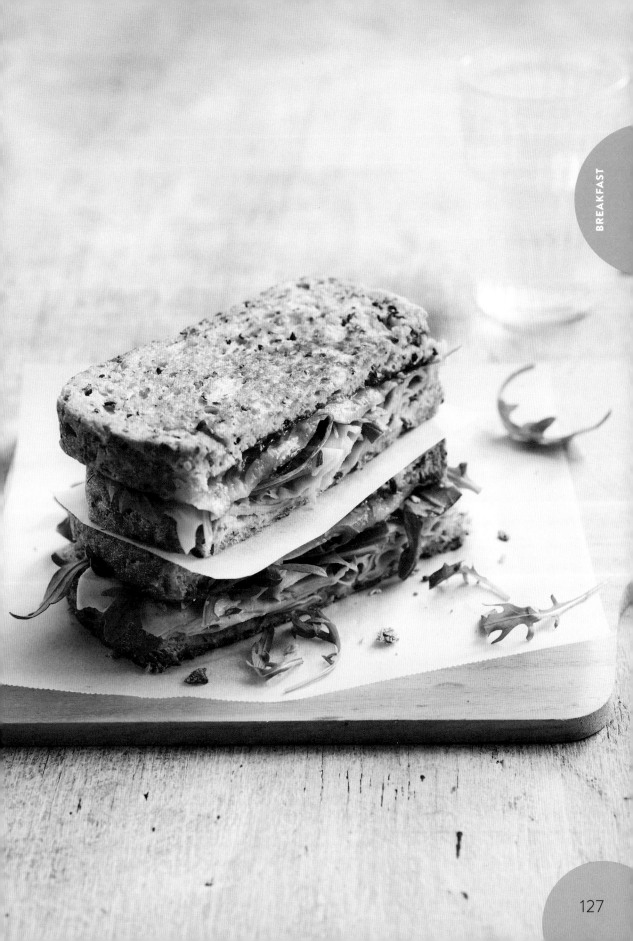

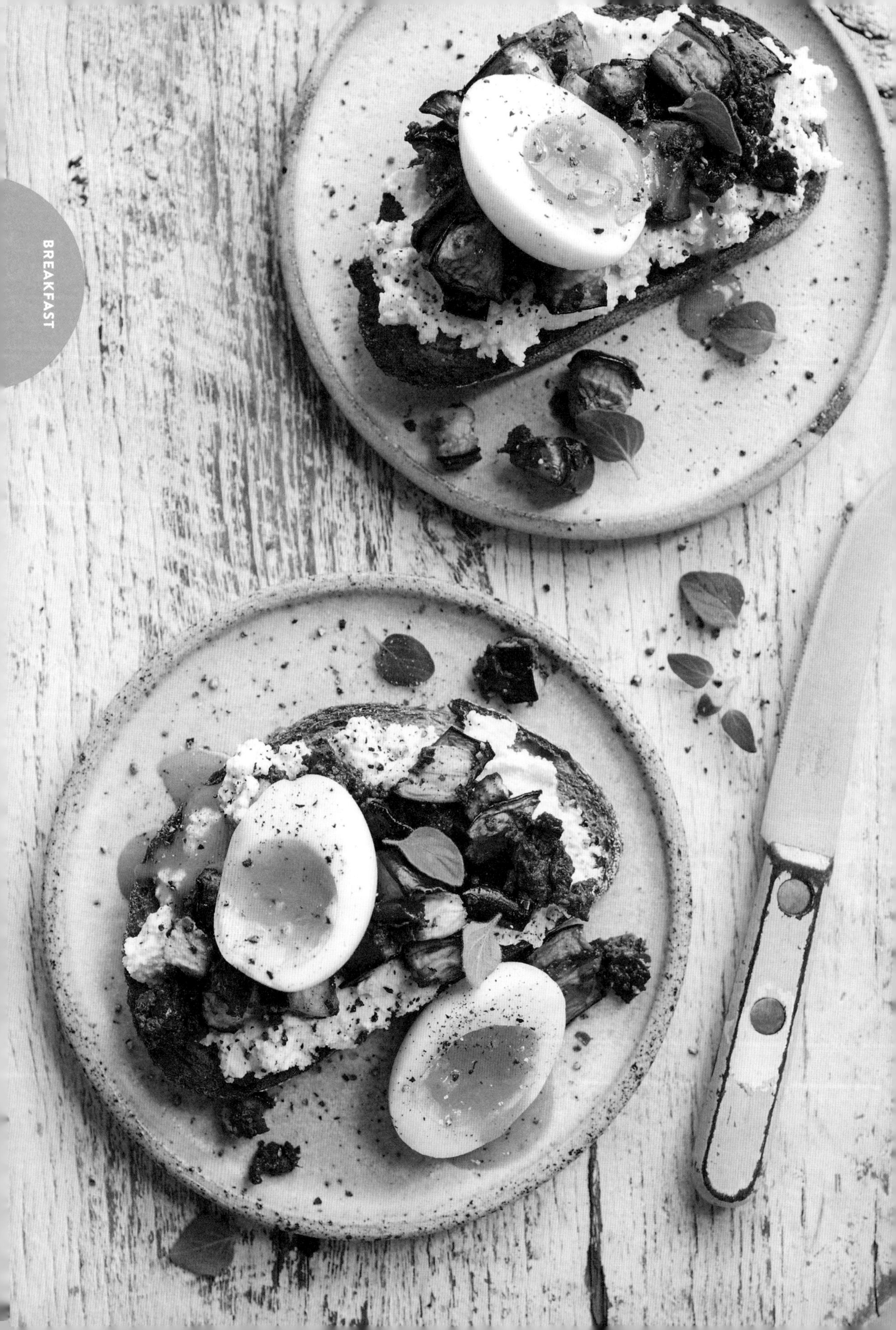

Ricotta, eggplant & olive bruschetta with soft-boiled eggs

Gone are the days when bruschetta was just the prelude to a main meal – this recipe puts it centre stage. The options for delicious toppings are endless. Forget soggy tomato bread: here is low-GI, nutritionally complete lusciousness. And the best part is that it's so simple, anyone can make this impressive weekend brunch.

SERVES 4 PREP TIME: 5 MINS COOKING TIME: 40 MINS

1 large eggplant (aubergine), diced
1 tablespoon olive oil
4 tablespoons olive tapenade
4 large eggs
4 slices rye sourdough or gluten-free
  wholegrain bread, toasted
250 g (9 oz) reduced-fat ricotta cheese

Preheat the oven to 180°C (350°F) fan-forced and line a baking tray with baking paper.

Place the eggplant on the tray, season with salt and pepper and brush with oil. Bake for 30 minutes until tender, then transfer to a bowl and toss with olive tapenade while the eggplant is still warm.

Meanwhile, put the eggs in a small saucepan of cold water and bring to the boil. When the water has boiled, remove from the heat and leave the eggs in the water for 2 minutes. Then run them under cold water and allow to cool slightly before peeling.

Spread ricotta cheese over each slice of toasted sourdough, spoon on the eggplant tapenade and top with a soft-boiled egg.

ANALYSIS SUMMARY

(PER SERVE) ENERGY 1119 KJ (268 CAL), PROTEIN 19 G, TOTAL FAT 9 G, SATURATED FAT 3 G, CARBOHYDRATE 24 G, SUGARS 7 G, DIETARY FIBRE 6 G

Za'atar-rolled eggs with beetroot & barley

Wholegrains such as barley are an important source of fibre and minerals. Barley is full of soluble fibre, which slows down digestion and delays sugar absorption into the bloodstream. This is what makes its glycaemic index so low, meaning it keeps you fuller for longer and provides you with steady energy. Za'atar is a great source of antioxidants. If you're gluten intolerant, you can substitute quinoa for the barley.

SERVES 4 PREP TIME: 5 MINS COOKING TIME: 40 MINS

2 cups (500 ml) salt-reduced vegetable stock
¾ cup (150 g) pearl barley
1 bunch English spinach, trimmed
8 eggs
3 tablespoons za'atar spice mix
1 large beetroot, peeled and grated
1 tablespoon pomegranate molasses
juice of 1 lemon
250 g (9 oz) smoked salmon

Put the stock in a small saucepan and bring to a simmer. Add the pearl barley, cover and simmer over low to medium heat for 30–35 minutes until the barley is tender and the liquid absorbed.

Bring a saucepan of water to the boil and blanch the spinach for 40 seconds. Remove and refresh in cold water.

Meanwhile, put the eggs in a small saucepan of cold water and bring to the boil. When the water has boiled, remove from the heat and leave the eggs in the water for 2 minutes. Then run them under cold water and allow to cool slightly before peeling.

Put the za'atar in a bowl; roll the eggs in the za'atar to coat.

While the barley is still warm, transfer it to a large bowl and stir through the beetroot, pomegranate molasses, lemon juice and spinach. Season with salt and pepper.

Spoon the barley mix into four bowls and place the smoked salmon and two za'atar eggs on top.

ANALYSIS SUMMARY

(PER SERVE) ENERGY 1509 KJ (359 CAL), PROTEIN 29 G, TOTAL FAT 10 G, SATURATED FAT 2 G, CARBOHYDRATE 33 G, SUGARS 9 G, DIETARY FIBRE 11 G

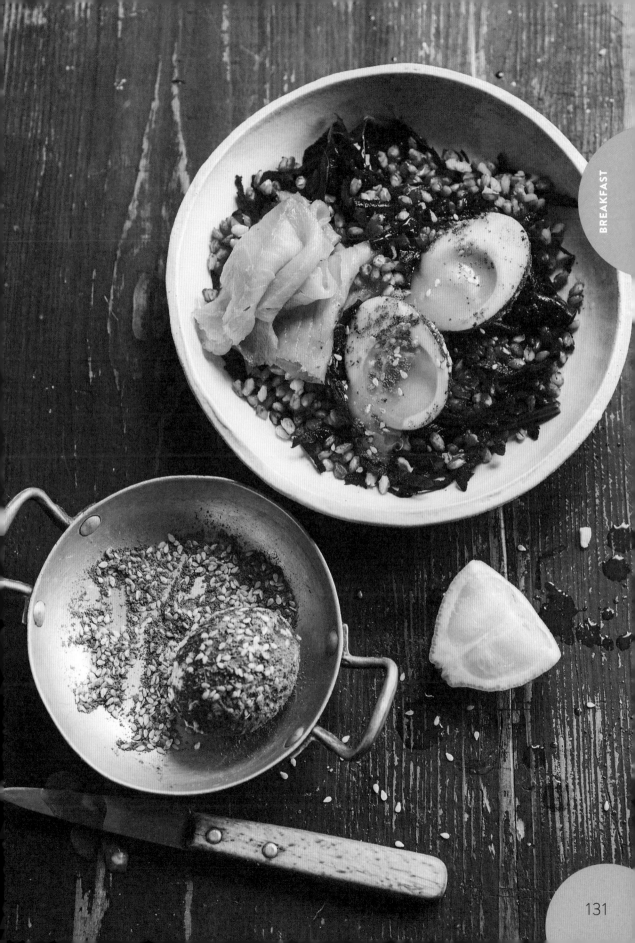

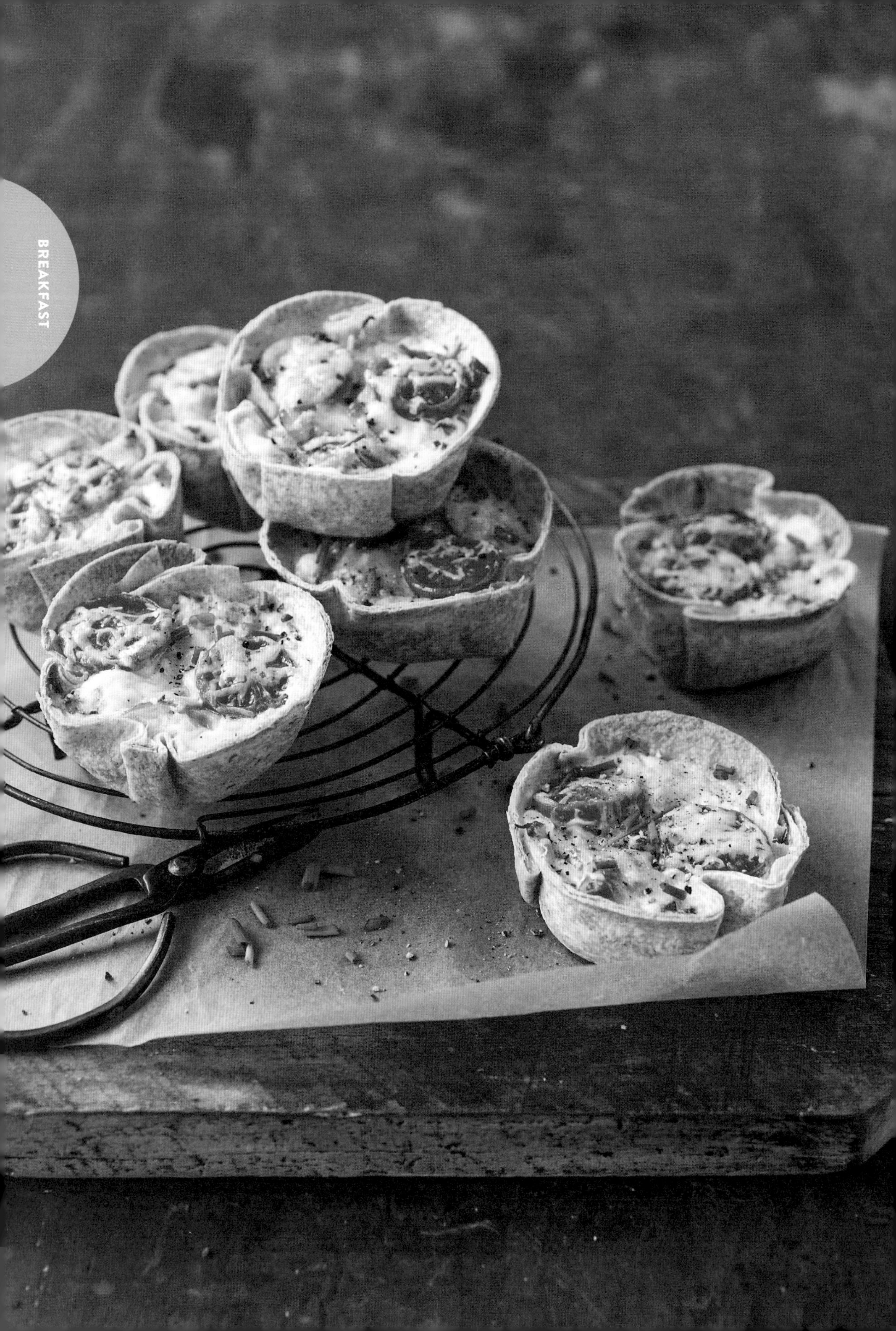

Ham, cheese & tomato mini breakfast quiches

Say goodbye to oily quiche Lorraine – these mini quiches are packed full of protein and low-GI carbs without all the saturated fat. They are ideal to make in advance and grab when you're running out the door in the morning, saving you from that impulsive bakery stop on the way to work. Good skin starts with good habits!

SERVES **4** PREP TIME: **10 MINS** COOKING TIME: **25 MINS**

4 wholemeal Lebanese flatbreads or gluten-free wraps
8 egg whites
⅓ cup (95 g) reduced-fat cottage cheese
3 tablespoons chopped chives
250 g (9 oz) leg ham, chopped
12 cherry tomatoes, halved
½ cup (50 g) grated parmesan cheese

Preheat the oven to 180°C (350°F) fan-forced and lightly grease 12 x ¾ cup (185 ml) muffin holes. With a 13 cm (5 inch) round cutter, cut three rounds from each flatbread. Push into the muffin holes.

Whisk together the egg whites, cottage cheese and chives. Stir in the ham and season with salt and pepper. Spoon into the muffin holes.

Place two cherry tomato halves on each quiche and scatter with parmesan. Bake for 25 minutes or until set.

ANALYSIS SUMMARY _____

(PER SERVE, 3 QUICHES) ENERGY 1524 KJ (364 CAL), PROTEIN 33 G, TOTAL FAT 8 G, SATURATED FAT 4 G, CARBOHYDRATE 35 G, SUGARS 4 G, DIETARY FIBRE 4 G

SNACKS
for great skin

Don't get caught with the between-meal munchies. This is when you are most likely to reach for quick pick-me-ups that are often high GI, high in salt and high in saturated fat. Arm yourself with simple snacks to stave off hunger, and also help you meet your fruit, veg, wholegrains, protein and dairy requirements for the day. This, in turn, will keep glucose and insulin levels steady and reduce sugar cravings. Here are some ideas that are easy to prepare, and that balance protein and low-GI carbohydrates to keep you looking and feeling great.

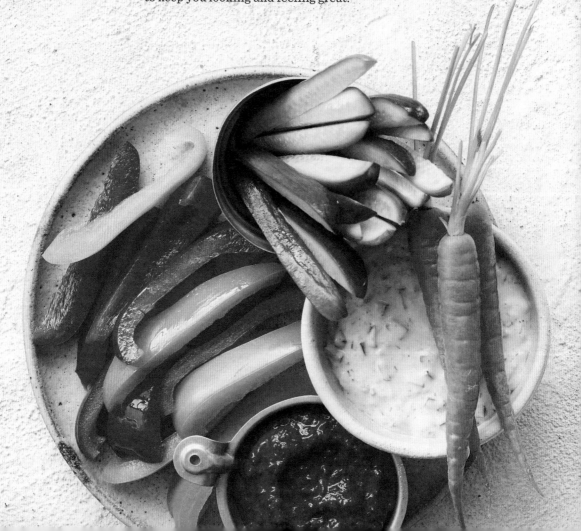

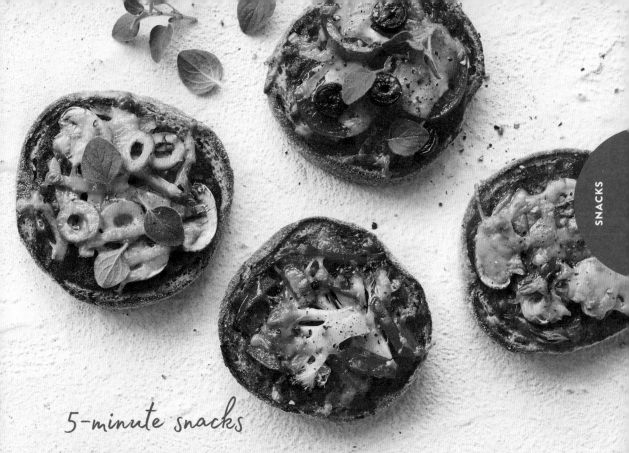

5-minute snacks

- Make **mini pizzas** with leftover meats, veggies and low-fat cheese toasted on wholegrain English muffins.
- Enjoy tinned **flavoured tuna in olive oil** with wholemeal crackers.
- Spread avocado and tomato, **ricotta and banana**, curried egg or vegemite and cottage cheese on wholemeal crackers.
- Make **tzatziki** — following the recipe on page 172 — and enjoy with vegetable sticks.
- Make **hummus** — made with chickpeas, tahini, garlic, lemon juice and olive oil, with added beetroot, if you like it.

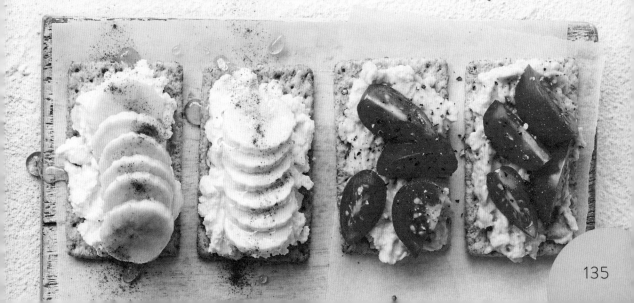

Roasted chickpeas

400 g (14 oz) tin chickpeas, rinsed
1 tablespoon olive oil
1 tablespoon spices or chopped herbs (such as curry powder,
    garam masala, cumin, smoked paprika, rosemary, thyme)

Preheat the oven to 180°C (350°F). Toss the chickpeas
in olive oil, spices or herbs and salt and pepper. Roast for
30 minutes until golden and crispy.

GLUTEN-FREE NIBBLES

These quick-and-easy snacks are so tasty that you won't
ever feel you are missing out. Low-GI carbohydrates
provide long-lasting energy and these snack plates also
contain plenty of fibre for your digestion.

Sweet potato chips

1 sweet potato, cut into chips
1 tablespoon olive oil
1 teaspoon cumin

Preheat the oven to 180°C (350°F). Toss the
sweet potato chips in the olive oil, cumin and some
salt and pepper. Bake for 20 minutes or until the
chips start to brown and crisp.

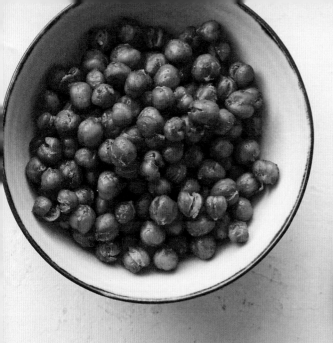
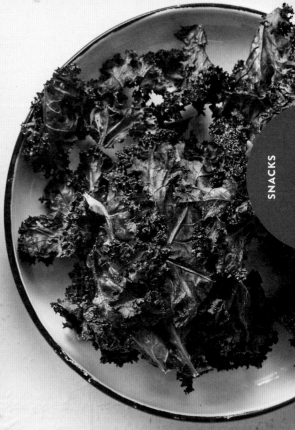

Kale chips

1 bunch kale leaves (stems cut out)
1 tablespoon olive oil
1 teaspoon paprika

Preheat the oven to 180°C (350°F). Tear the kale leaves into
bite-sized pieces and toss in olive oil, paprika and salt and pepper.
Bake for 15–20 minutes or until crisp.

Super-simple gluten-free snacks

- **Trail mix** — mix together raw unsalted nuts (walnuts, almonds or
  brazil nuts), seeds (sunflower seeds, pepitas or flaxseeds/linseeds)
  and dried fruit (sultanas, raisins, apricots, cranberries or goji berries).
- **Protein balls** — make a stash of Fig and brazil nut bombs from
  page 224.
- **Popcorn** — toss with olive oil instead of butter, and add herbs
  and spices to keep it interesting.

5-minute fruities

- **Frozen yoghurt blueberries**: dip blueberries in yoghurt and spread on baking paper to freeze overnight.
- **Apple slices** and almond butter.
- **Banana and peanut butter** on toasted wholemeal pitta bread.
- **Fruit smoothies**: experiment with different fruits and greens. Use the recipes on pages 102 and 105 as a base.

FRUITY SNACKS

Packed with antioxidants, vitamin C, fibre and energy, combined with protein, these snacks will help protect your skin and give you a pick-me-up when you're feeling sluggish.

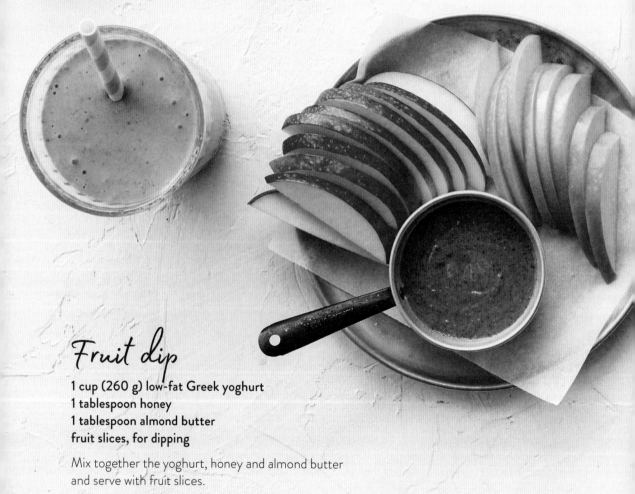

Fruit dip

1 cup (260 g) low-fat Greek yoghurt
1 tablespoon honey
1 tablespoon almond butter
fruit slices, for dipping

Mix together the yoghurt, honey and almond butter and serve with fruit slices.

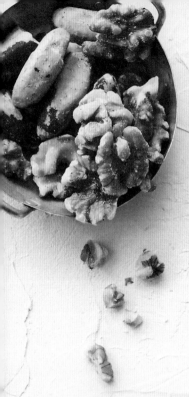

Parfait your way

Confused about which yoghurt to choose? You're not alone. Low-fat natural or Greek yoghurt is the perfect snack – it's high in protein, low-GI carbohydrate and probiotics for gut health and digestion, but you might be bored of the flavour? Commercial fancy flavoured yoghurts can be high in fat and added sugar and low in good bacteria, providing little nutrition.

I have a solution. Yoghurt parfaits are a great way to tart up low-fat Greek yoghurt with exciting textures and flavours.

PICK YOUR YOGHURT:

¾ cup (200 g) low-fat natural yoghurt (mild light flavour)
¾ cup (200 g) low-fat Greek yoghurt
 (creamy and tangy)

SPRINKLE WITH TOPPINGS:

- Chopped fruit
- Natural muesli
- Puffed rice (GF)
- Quinoa flakes (GF)
- Cacao nibs
- Bee pollen (from health food shops)
- Chopped nuts (almonds, walnuts, brazil nuts)
- Seeds (flaxseeds/linseeds, pepitas/pumpkin seeds, sunflower seeds, chia seeds)

- Buckwheat (GF)
- Honey (just 2 teaspoons)
- Protein powder (for a little sweetness and extra protein)

Eat straightaway or secure with a lid and refrigerate for later.

Not fruit... but dairylicious

You can't beat a glass of cold milk. It provides the perfect balance of protein and low-GI carbohydrate. If you're drinking milk substitutes, make sure they're calcium fortified and contain no added sugar.

Curried chicken & mango salad : GF

Rethink how you reach your two fruit serves a day with this showstopper! Sweet mango, peppery rocket, creamy avocado and savoury spices make this perfectly balanced dish a no-brainer. It's packed full of prebiotics for a healthy gut, vitamin C for collagen production and monounsaturated fats for cell hydration and insulation. Yoghurt is used as a clever alternative to mayonnaise, which can be high in saturated fat, sugar and preservatives.

SERVES **4** PREP TIME: **15 MINS** COOKING TIME: **20 MINS**

500 g (1 lb 2 oz) chicken breasts
1 teaspoon olive oil
1 teaspoon curry powder
100 g (3½ oz) green beans, topped
    and tailed
3 cups (105 g) rocket (arugula)
½ red onion, finely sliced
1 Lebanese cucumber, sliced

2 mangoes, flesh chopped
1 small avocado, chopped

DRESSING
grated zest and juice of 1 lime
4 tablespoons low-fat Greek yoghurt
2 tablespoons good-quality mango chutney
1 teaspoon curry powder

Preheat the oven to 180°C (350°F) fan-forced and line a baking tray with foil.

Put the chicken on the tray and rub with the oil and curry powder, then season with salt and pepper. Bake for 20 minutes. Set aside to rest for 5 minutes, then slice.

Meanwhile, bring a small saucepan of water to the boil and blanch the green beans for 2–3 minutes until bright green and tender yet crisp. Refresh under cold running water. Drain.

To make the dressing, combine all the ingredients in a small bowl.

Combine the rocket, onion, green beans, cucumber and mango in a large bowl. Toss with half the dressing.

Transfer the salad to a large serving platter. Scatter with avocado, lay the chicken slices on top and drizzle with the remaining dressing. Serve with a squeeze of lime juice.

ANALYSIS SUMMARY

(PER SERVE) ENERGY 1544 KJ (370 CAL) , PROTEIN 34 G, TOTAL FAT 9 G, SATURATED FAT 2 G, CARBOHYDRATE 32 G, SUGARS 32 G, DIETARY FIBRE 6 G

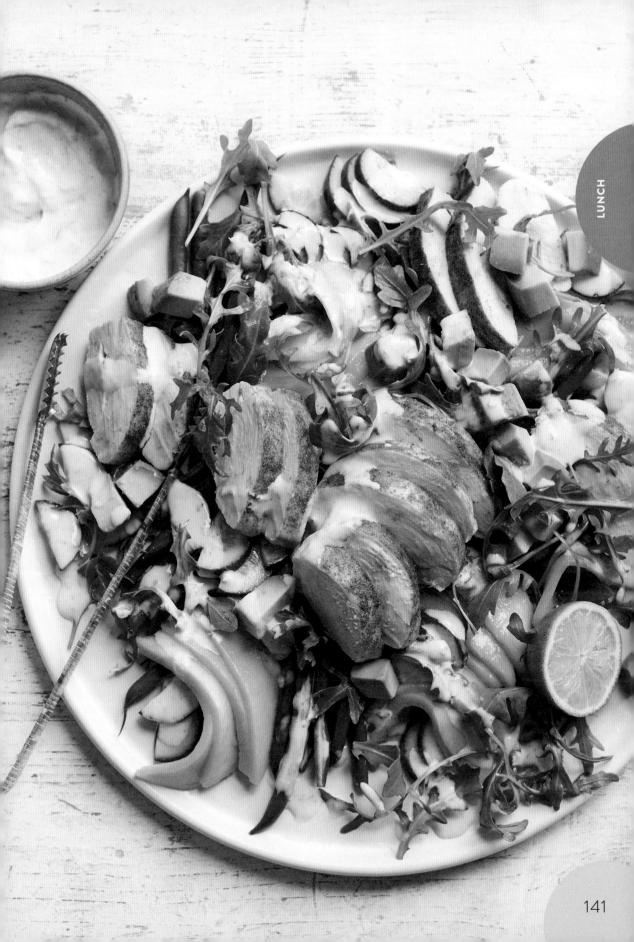

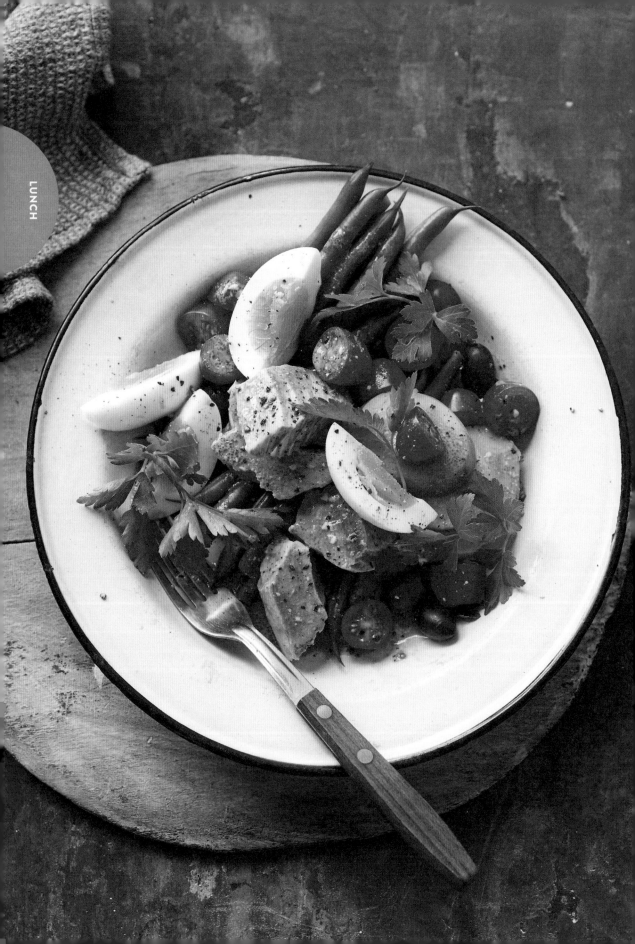

Tuna niçoise salad : GF

This classic Mediterranean meal contains all the good things. It's gluten free and boasts low-GI carbohydrates, lean protein and healthy fat: a win–win for your skin and a happy, healthy body.

SERVES **2** PREP TIME: **10 MINS** COOKING TIME: **25 MINS**

3 pontiac potatoes
200 g (7 oz) green beans, topped and tailed
2 eggs
1 tablespoon olive oil
2 tablespoons red wine vinegar
2 teaspoons dijon mustard

¼ teaspoon caster sugar
150 g (5½ oz) tuna steaks or tinned tuna, drained
250 g (9 oz) cherry tomatoes, halved
½ cup (60 g) pitted black olives
½ handful chopped flat-leaf parsley

Cook the potatoes in boiling water for 10 minutes or until just tender. Use a slotted spoon to transfer the potatoes to a chopping board, then cut each one in half. Add the green beans to the saucepan and cook for 2–3 minutes until bright green and tender yet crisp. Refresh under cold running water. Drain.

Meanwhile, put the eggs in a saucepan of cold water. Bring to the boil over high heat. Reduce the heat to simmer for 6–7 minutes. Drain and cool under cold running water. Peel and quarter.

To make a dressing, whisk together the oil, vinegar, mustard and sugar in a jug. Season with salt and pepper.

If you're using tuna steaks, heat a frying pan over medium–high heat. Add the tuna and cook for 2–3 minutes on each side for medium or longer if you prefer. Set aside for 5 minutes to rest and then flake the tuna into large pieces.

Spoon the potato, green beans, egg, tuna, tomato, olives and parsley into bowls. Drizzle with the dressing and season before serving.

ANALYSIS SUMMARY

(PER SERVE) ENERGY 1821 KJ (436 CAL), PROTEIN 33 G, TOTAL FAT 16 G, SATURATED FAT 3 G, CARBOHYDRATE 34 G, SUGARS 5 G, DIETARY FIBRE 7 G

Moroccan chickpea salad : GF

If you're an omnivore, eating vegetarian occasionally can be a great way to add variety to your weekly menu. It's important to think about combining different sources of protein to ensure you're obtaining all the essential amino acids. This recipe features chickpeas, boiled eggs and yoghurt to bump up the amino acid profile; these ingredients also add some interesting textures.

SERVES 2 PREP TIME: **10 MINS** COOKING TIME: **5 MINS**

2 teaspoons olive oil
200 g (7 oz) tinned chickpeas,
   drained and rinsed
1 cup (125 g) small cauliflower florets
1 teaspoon ground cumin
1 garlic clove, crushed
1 carrot, peeled into ribbons
3 tablespoons currants

1 spring onion (scallion), chopped
2 eggs
1 tablespoon sunflower seeds

DRESSING
⅓ cup (95 g) low-fat Greek yoghurt
2 teaspoons tahini
2 tablespoons lemon juice

Heat the oil in a non-stick frying pan over medium heat. Add the chickpeas, cauliflower, cumin and garlic. Cook, stirring often, for 5 minutes. Remove from the heat and tip into a large bowl.

Add the carrot, currants and spring onion to the bowl.

Meanwhile, put the eggs in a small saucepan of cold water and bring to the boil. When the water has boiled, remove from the heat and leave the eggs in the water for 2 minutes. Then run them under cold water and allow to cool slightly before peeling.

To make the dressing, whisk together all the ingredients.

To serve, drizzle the dressing over the salad. Top with the soft-boiled eggs and sunflower seeds.

ANALYSIS SUMMARY ─────────────────────────────

(PER SERVE) ENERGY 1424 KJ (345 CAL), PROTEIN 19 G, TOTAL FAT 11 G, SATURATED FAT 2 G, CARBOHYDRATE 34 G, SUGARS 20 G, DIETARY FIBRE 12 G

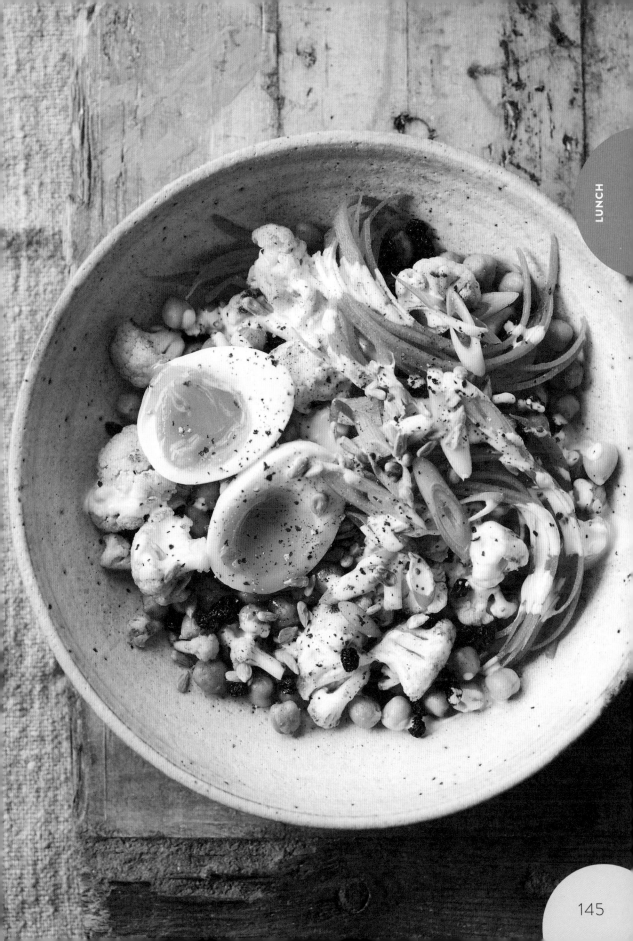

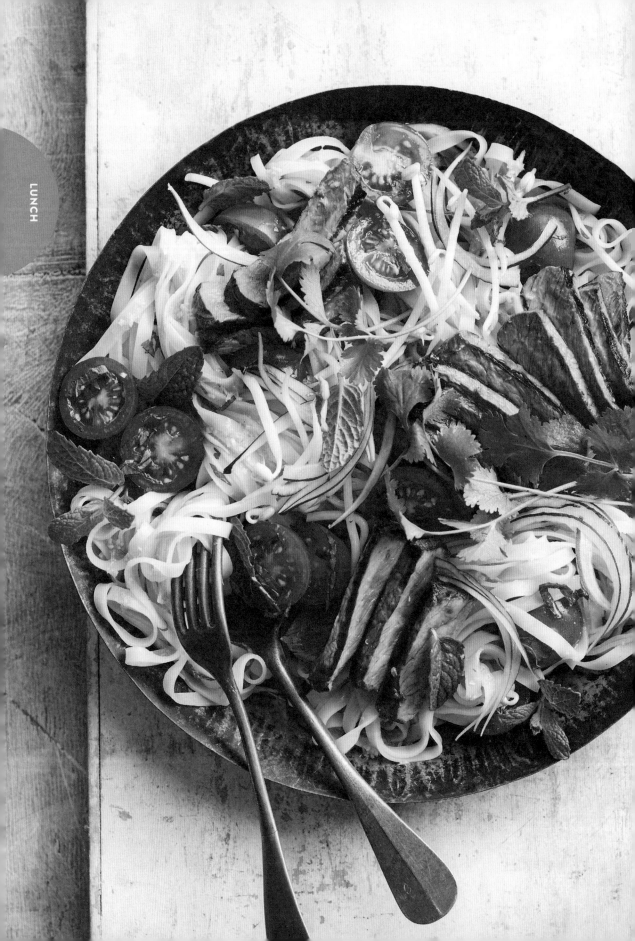

Thai beef noodle salad : GF

Using rice noodles makes this dish gluten free and perfect as a light and fresh lunch or even dinner. I find a common misconception is that red meat should be avoided because it is high in saturated fat and therefore bad for your health, but lean cuts of beef are an excellent source of iron, which is particularly important for women. An adequate iron intake ensures sufficient oxygen in the blood, which gives us lots of energy and a healthy glow. You'll find lemongrass paste next to the fresh herb section in the supermarket.

SERVES **4** PREP TIME: **15 MINS** COOKING TIME: **15 MINS**

150 g (5½ oz) rice stick noodles
500 g (1 lb 2 oz) lean rump steak
250 g (9 oz) cherry tomatoes, cut in half
1 cup (115 g) bean sprouts
½ red onion, sliced
1 handful chopped coriander (cilantro)
1 handful chopped mint

DRESSING
3 tablespoons lemon juice
1 tablespoon fish sauce
2 teaspoons lemongrass paste

Cook the noodles in a saucepan of boiling water for 4–5 minutes until tender. Drain, then rinse under cold water.

Heat a chargrill pan over medium–high heat. Cook the steak for 3–4 minutes on each side for medium or until cooked to your liking. Transfer to a plate and cover loosely with foil. Set aside for 5 minutes to rest. Slice thinly.

Whisk together the dressing ingredients.

Put the noodles in a bowl and add the cherry tomatoes, bean sprouts, onion, coriander, mint and half the dressing. Toss gently.

Top with the sliced beef and serve with the remaining dressing.

ANALYSIS SUMMARY _____

(PER SERVE) ENERGY 1498 KJ (358 CAL), PROTEIN 33 G, TOTAL FAT 7 G, SATURATED FAT 2 G, CARBOHYDRATE 35 G, SUGARS 5 G, DIETARY FIBRE 6 G

Vietnamese chicken salad pitta

Your body will thank you for this salad – it's the freshest of the fresh. It's always wise to check for hidden amounts of added sugar in shop-bought Asian sauces and dressings. You could be eating an additional seven to 10 teaspoons of sugar and not even know it. Ready-made dressings are handy when you're rushing to save time, but taking a few extra minutes to make your own (or look for a low-sugar dressing) could save your skin.

SERVES **4** PREP TIME: **10 MINS** COOKING TIME: **10 MINS**

400 g (14 oz) chicken breasts
¼ Chinese cabbage (wong bok), chopped
2 carrots, peeled and cut into matchsticks
1 red capsicum (pepper), seeded and sliced into thin strips
1 handful mint, chopped
1 handful coriander (cilantro), chopped
½ cup (70 g) peanuts, chopped
2 wholegrain pitta breads, pockets or gluten-free wraps

DRESSING
3 tablespoons fish sauce
3 tablespoons rice wine vinegar
2 teaspoons honey
1 garlic clove, crushed
1 red chilli, seeded and finely chopped
2 tablespoons lime juice

Put the chicken in a saucepan, cover with cold water and bring to the boil. Reduce the heat to low and simmer for 10 minutes or until cooked through. Remove from the pan and rest for 5 minutes before shredding.

To make the dressing, whisk all the ingredients together.

Put the cabbage, carrot, capsicum, mint, coriander and chicken in a large bowl. Add the dressing and toss to combine. Sprinkle with the peanuts.

To serve, cut the breads in half and fill with the chicken salad.

ANALYSIS SUMMARY

(PER SERVE) ENERGY 1572 KJ (376 CAL), PROTEIN 28 G, TOTAL FAT 13 G, SATURATED FAT 3 G, CARBOHYDRATE 31 G, SUGARS 25 G, DIETARY FIBRE 10 G

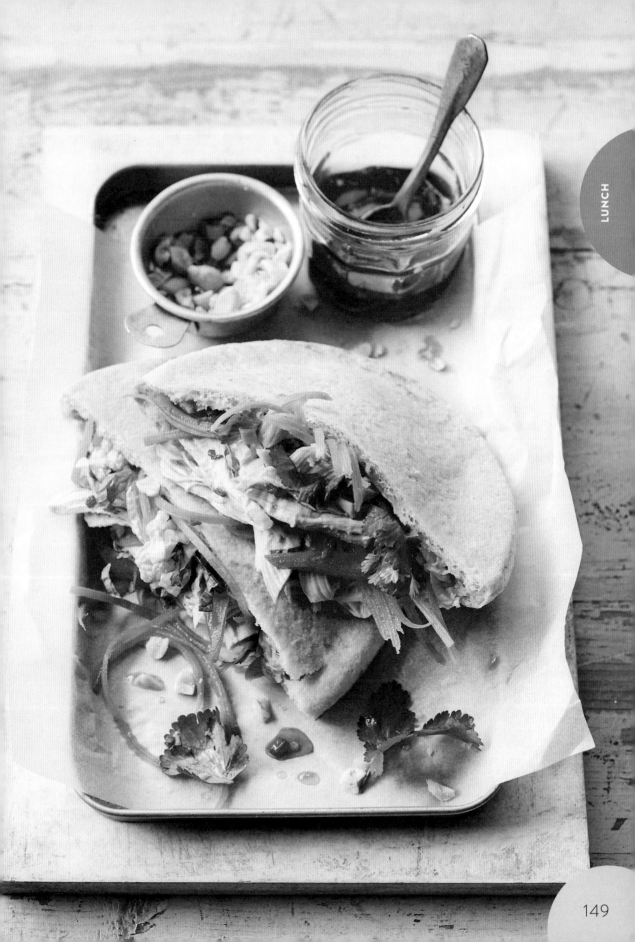

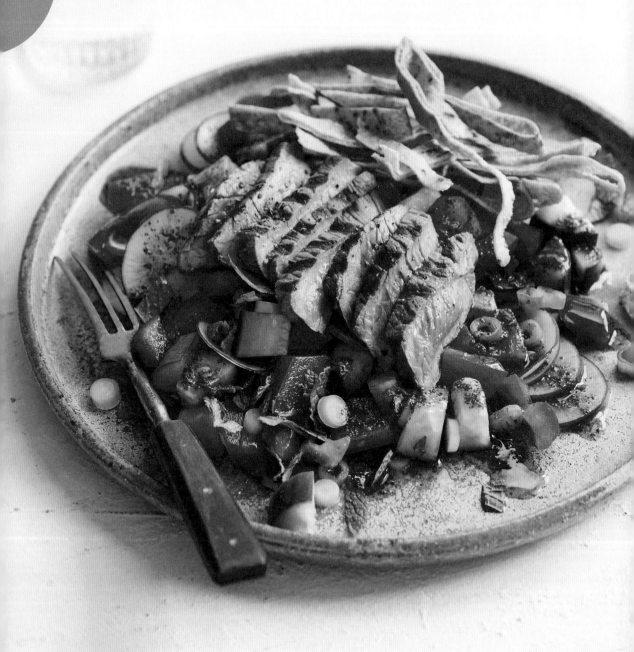

Lamb fattoush

Lamb is a great source of protein and iron but it can be high in saturated fat, so I always look for the leaner cuts of meat. I also aim for two to three serves of lean red meat per week, to ensure an adequate iron intake.

SERVES **4** PREP TIME: **10 MINS** COOKING TIME: **10 MINS**

3 wholemeal Lebanese flatbreads or gluten-free wraps, sliced into 1 cm strips
2 tomatoes, chopped
2 Lebanese cucumbers, chopped
1 red capsicum (pepper), seeded and chopped
4 radishes, sliced into rounds
2 spring onions (scallions), chopped

1 handful mint, coarsely chopped
450 g (1 lb) lean lamb steaks

DRESSING
3 tablespoons lemon juice
2 tablespoons olive oil
1 garlic clove, crushed
1 tablespoons sumac

Preheat the oven to 180°C (350°F) fan-forced and line a baking tray with baking paper. Put the flatbread strips on the tray and bake for 5 minutes or until golden and crunchy.

In a large bowl, mix together the tomato, cucumber, capsicum, radish, spring onion and mint.

Mix together all the dressing ingredients. Drizzle over the salad and toss to combine.

Preheat a chargrill pan over medium–high heat. Add the lamb steaks and cook for 3 minutes each side for medium or to your liking. Transfer to a plate and cover with foil for 5 minutes, then slice.

Serve the salad in bowls, topped with the lamb slices and the crunchy flatbread strips.

ANALYSIS SUMMARY ─────────────────────────────

(PER SERVE) ENERGY 1729 KJ (414 CAL), PROTEIN 32 G, TOTAL FAT 16 G, SATURATED FAT 3 G, CARBOHYDRATE 31 G, SUGARS 7 G, DIETARY FIBRE 7 G

Quinoa, broccoli & haloumi salad with green goddess dressing : GF

If you avoid salads because you think they're boring, you've been doing it all wrong. You don't need to be vegetarian to love this recipe. It's every superfood rolled into one delicious bowl of nourishment, full of prebiotics for a healthy gut microbiome and antioxidants to protect the skin from free-radical damage.

SERVES **4** PREP TIME: **20 MINS** COOKING TIME: **20 MINS**

1 cup (200 g) quinoa
1 head (about 400 g) broccoli, chopped
   into small florets
2 zucchini (courgettes), peeled into ribbons
4 eggs
3 cups (105 g) rocket (arugula)
150 g (5½ oz) haloumi cheese, sliced
pomegranate seeds

GREEN GODDESS DRESSING
¼ avocado
3 tablespoons white wine vinegar
1 spring onion (scallion), chopped
1 handful coriander (cilantro) leaves,
   chopped
3 tablespoons low-fat Greek yoghurt
1 garlic clove, crushed

Rinse the quinoa, put it in a saucepan with 2 cups (500 ml) of water and bring to the boil. Reduce the heat to medium, cover the pan and cook for 15 minutes or until tender. Drain and return to the pan. Stir in the broccoli and zucchini and let them cook in the residual heat.

Meanwhile, put the eggs in a small saucepan of cold water and bring to the boil. Reduce the heat to simmer for 6–7 minutes, then remove the eggs with a slotted spoon, run them under cold water and allow to cool slightly before peeling.

To make the dressing, put all the ingredients in a small food processor. Blend until smooth and season with salt and pepper.

Combine the broccoli and zucchini quinoa with the rocket and eggs and spoon into bowls.

Heat a large dry frying pan (no need to add oil) and cook the haloumi for 1 minute on each side or until golden.

Top the salad bowls with haloumi and pomegranate seeds. Serve with the dressing on the side.

ANALYSIS SUMMARY

(PER SERVE) ENERGY 1810 KJ (431 CAL), PROTEIN 31 G, TOTAL FAT 15 G, SATURATED FAT 6 G, CARBOHYDRATE 34 G, SUGARS 10 G, DIETARY FIBRE 12 G

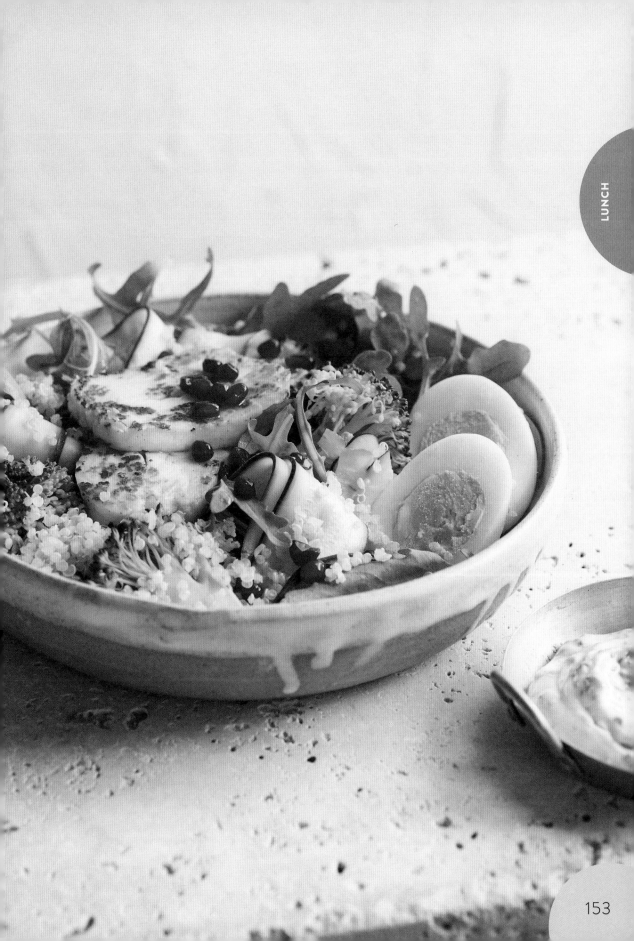

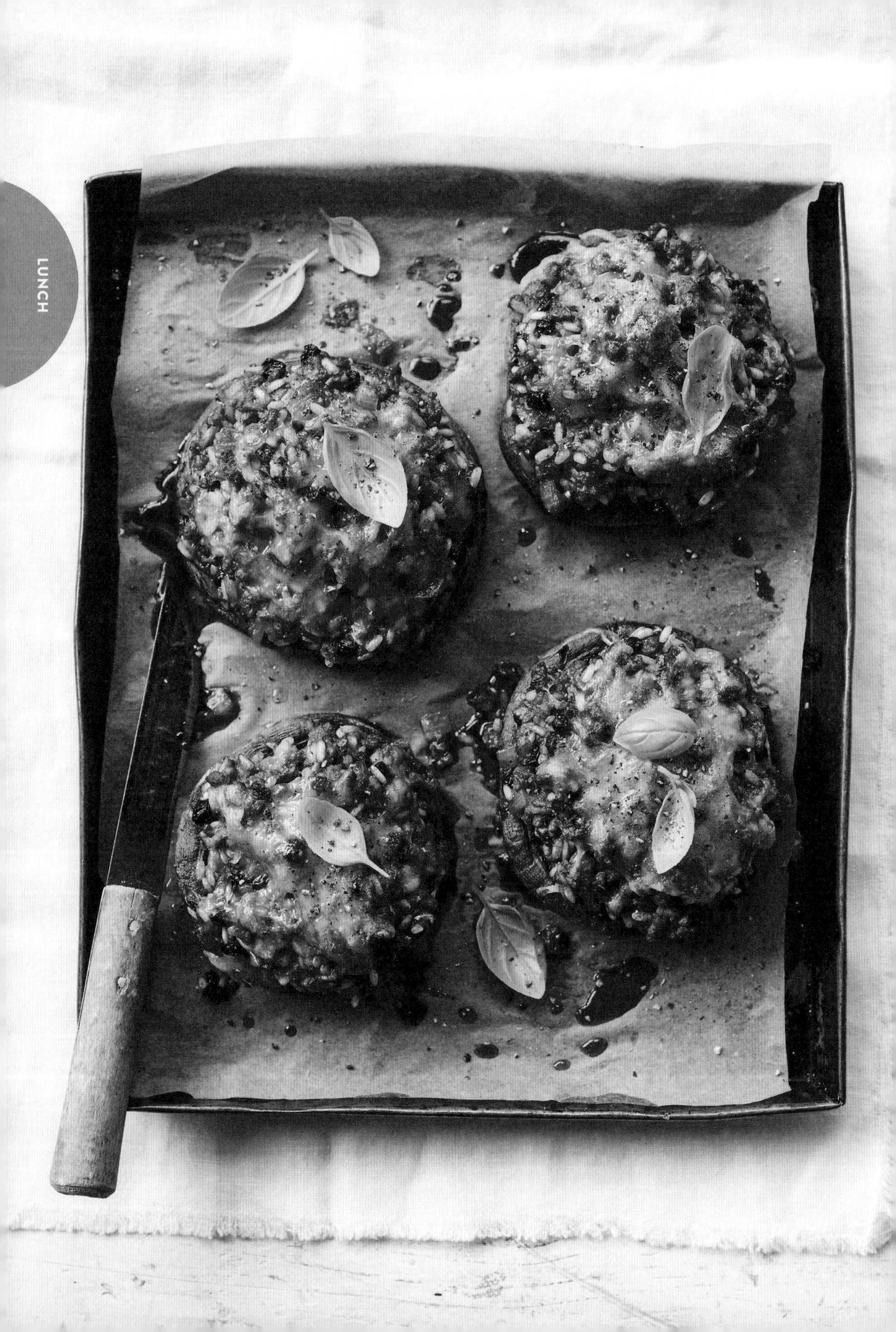

Stuffed mushrooms : GF

These are fabulous savoury, sweet, herbaceous, cheesy mounds of goodness. A few simple swaps transform this dish into a well-balanced, healthy lunch that's low in fat, low GI and high in protein. This could become your new go-to lunch (although I love to eat these for breakfast, too).

SERVES 4 PREP TIME: 10 MINS COOKING TIME: 1 HOUR

1 tablespoon olive oil
400 g (14 oz) lean minced beef
1 brown onion, chopped
2 garlic cloves, crushed
400 g (14 oz) tin chopped tomatoes
1 teaspoon cumin seeds
1½ cups (375 ml) salt-reduced beef stock
½ cup (100 g) brown rice
½ cup (75 g) currants
1 handful basil leaves, chopped
4 large field mushrooms, stems removed
½ cup (50 g) grated reduced-fat cheddar cheese

Preheat the oven to 180°C (350°F) fan-forced.

Heat the oil in a large frying pan over medium heat and add the mince, onion and garlic. Fry for 5–10 minutes until the mince is just browned. Add the tomatoes, cumin seeds and stock. Cook for 5 minutes, then add the rice and reduce the heat to low. Simmer for 25 minutes, stirring often, or until the rice is tender and liquid has thickened. Stir in the currants and basil.

Put the mushrooms gill-side up in a baking dish and fill with the beef and rice mixture. Scatter with cheddar cheese.

Bake for 20–30 minutes until the cheese is golden brown and the mushrooms are cooked through.

ANALYSIS SUMMARY _____

(PER SERVE) ENERGY 1724 KJ (412 CAL), PROTEIN 34 G, TOTAL FAT 14 G, SATURATED FAT 6 G, CARBOHYDRATE 32 G, SUGARS 11 G, DIETARY FIBRE 7 G

Warm salmon & potato salad with sauerkraut : GF

This recipe is perfect for using up leftover salmon fillet from the night before, or as a last-minute pantry meal using tinned salmon. Both are full of omega-3 fats for healthy skin. Salty, sour, crunchy sauerkraut is a natural probiotic that makes healthy tummies, which make healthy skin – so eat up.

SERVES 4 PREP TIME: **10 MINS** COOKING TIME: **20 MINS**

800 g (1 lb 12 oz) baby potatoes, cut in half
300 g (10½ oz) green beans, topped and tailed
3 Lebanese cucumbers, sliced
2 spring onions (scallions), chopped
¾ cup (115 g) sauerkraut
500 g (1 lb 2 oz) leftover grilled salmon, flaked,
   or tinned red salmon

DRESSING
¾ cup (200 g) low-fat Greek yoghurt
juice of 1 lemon
1 tablespoon dijon mustard
2 teaspoons honey

Put the potatoes in a large saucepan, cover with cold water and bring to the boil. Reduce the heat to simmer for 10–15 minutes until tender but still holding their shape. Drain and transfer to a bowl.

Meanwhile, blanch the green beans for 2–3 minutes in boiling water until bright green and tender yet crisp. Refresh under cold water.

Combine all the dressing ingredients and season with salt and pepper.

While the potatoes are still warm, toss with the green beans, cucumber, spring onion and sauerkraut.

Gently stir in the salmon and drizzle with the dressing.

ANALYSIS SUMMARY _____

(PER SERVE) ENERGY 1582 KJ (378 CAL), PROTEIN 39 G, TOTAL FAT 8 G, SATURATED FAT 2 G, CARBOHYDRATE 33 G, SUGARS 11 G, DIETARY FIBRE 6 G

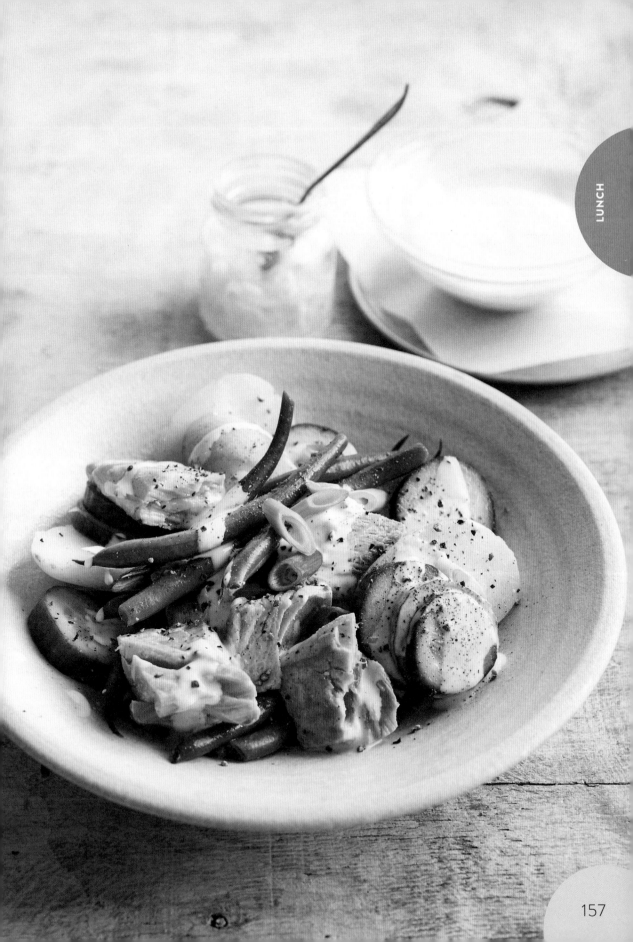

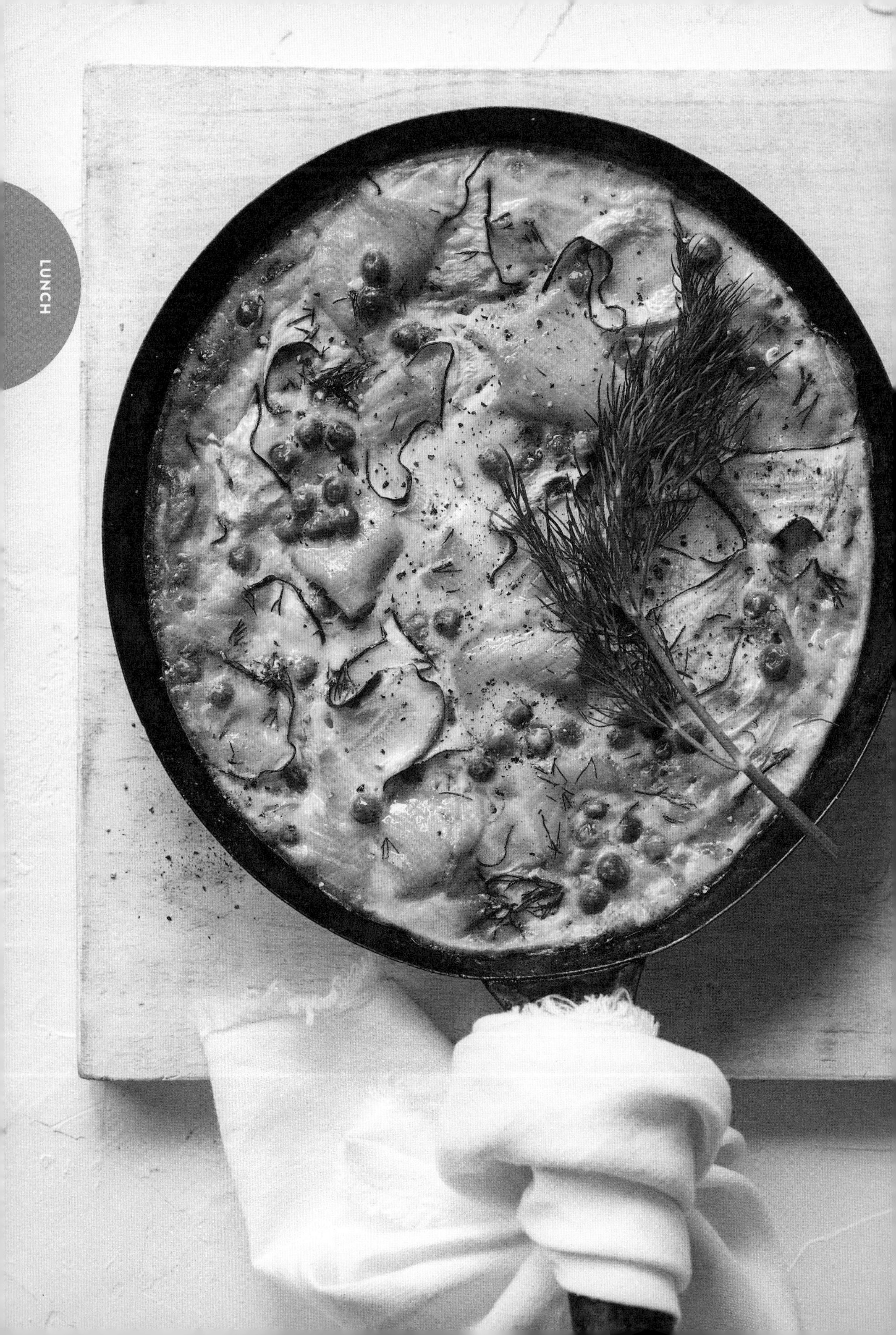

Salmon, dill & zucchini frittata : GF

This no-fuss, gluten-free frittata is high in omega-3, protein and vegetables – perfect for nourishing lunches on the go. You can use up any seasonal vegetables in your fridge crisper to create a cheap, throw-together meal. The frittata is just as good hot out of the oven or cold the next day: you really can't go wrong.

SERVES **2** PREP TIME: **10 MINS** COOKING TIME: **25 MINS**

1 teaspoon olive oil
2 potatoes, thinly sliced into rounds
3 eggs plus 3 extra egg whites
1 handful dill, chopped
1 cup (140 g) peas
1 zucchini (courgette), shaved into ribbons
100 g (3½ oz) smoked salmon, chopped

Heat the oil in an ovenproof frying pan over medium heat. Add the potatoes in a single layer and cook for 4–5 minutes on each side.

Whisk together the eggs, egg whites and dill. Add the peas, zucchini and smoked salmon. Season well with salt and pepper.

Preheat the grill to medium–high.

Pour the egg mixture over the potatoes in the pan and cook for 5 minutes or until the base of the frittata starts to set.

Place the pan under the grill for a further 10 minutes or until the frittata has risen and started to brown on top.

The frittata can be served immediately, or you can leave it to cool and then refrigerate it to eat later (it will keep for 1 day).

ANALYSIS SUMMARY

(PER SERVE) ENERGY 1526 KJ (364 CAL), PROTEIN 33 G, TOTAL FAT 10 G, SATURATED FAT 2 G, CARBOHYDRATE 31 G, SUGARS 7 G, DIETARY FIBRE 8 G

Tuna poke bowl

Nourishing, fresh and wholesome, it's no wonder poke bowls are all the rage. If you can't find sashimi-grade tuna, buy a fillet of tuna and cook it to your liking or use good-quality tinned tuna. Kimchi is a spicy and sour Korean condiment made from fermented vegetables. Research indicates that *Lactobacillus* bacteria in kimchi may help reduce inflammation and even dermatitis. You can use tamari or gluten-free soy here if you're gluten intolerant.

SERVES 2 PREP TIME: **10 MINS** COOKING TIME: **25 MINS**

½ cup (100 g) brown rice, rinsed
¼ red cabbage, shredded
1 cup (150 g) edamame beans
4 radishes, thinly sliced
1 tablespoon pickled ginger
2 tablespoons Korean kimchi
1 tablespoon salt-reduced soy sauce
150 g (5½ oz) sashimi-grade tuna, thinly sliced
lemon wedges, to serve
wasabi, to serve

Bring 4 cups (1 litre) of water to the boil in a saucepan. Add the rice and stir gently, then reduce the heat to a simmer and cook for 25 minutes until tender. Drain well and spoon into two bowls.

Mix together the cabbage, edamame, radish, ginger, kimchi and soy sauce and spoon over the rice.

Arrange the tuna slices on top and serve with a wedge of lemon and a little wasabi.

ANALYSIS SUMMARY ⎯⎯⎯⎯⎯⎯⎯⎯⎯⎯⎯⎯⎯⎯⎯⎯⎯⎯⎯⎯⎯⎯

(PER SERVE) ENERGY 1526 KJ (364 CAL), PROTEIN 33 G, TOTAL FAT 10 G, SATURATED FAT 2 G, CARBOHYDRATE 31 G, SUGARS 4 G, DIETARY FIBRE 8 G

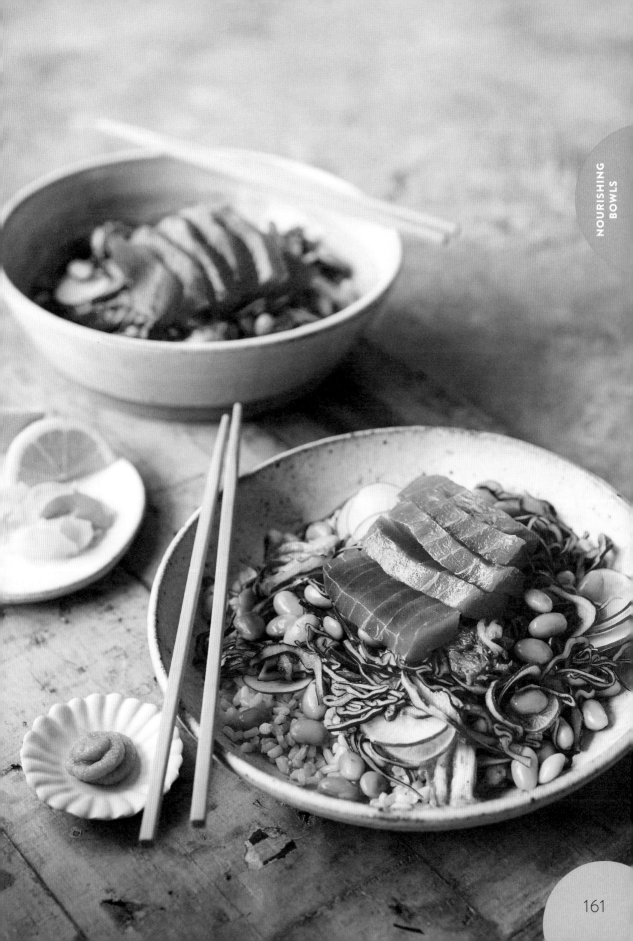

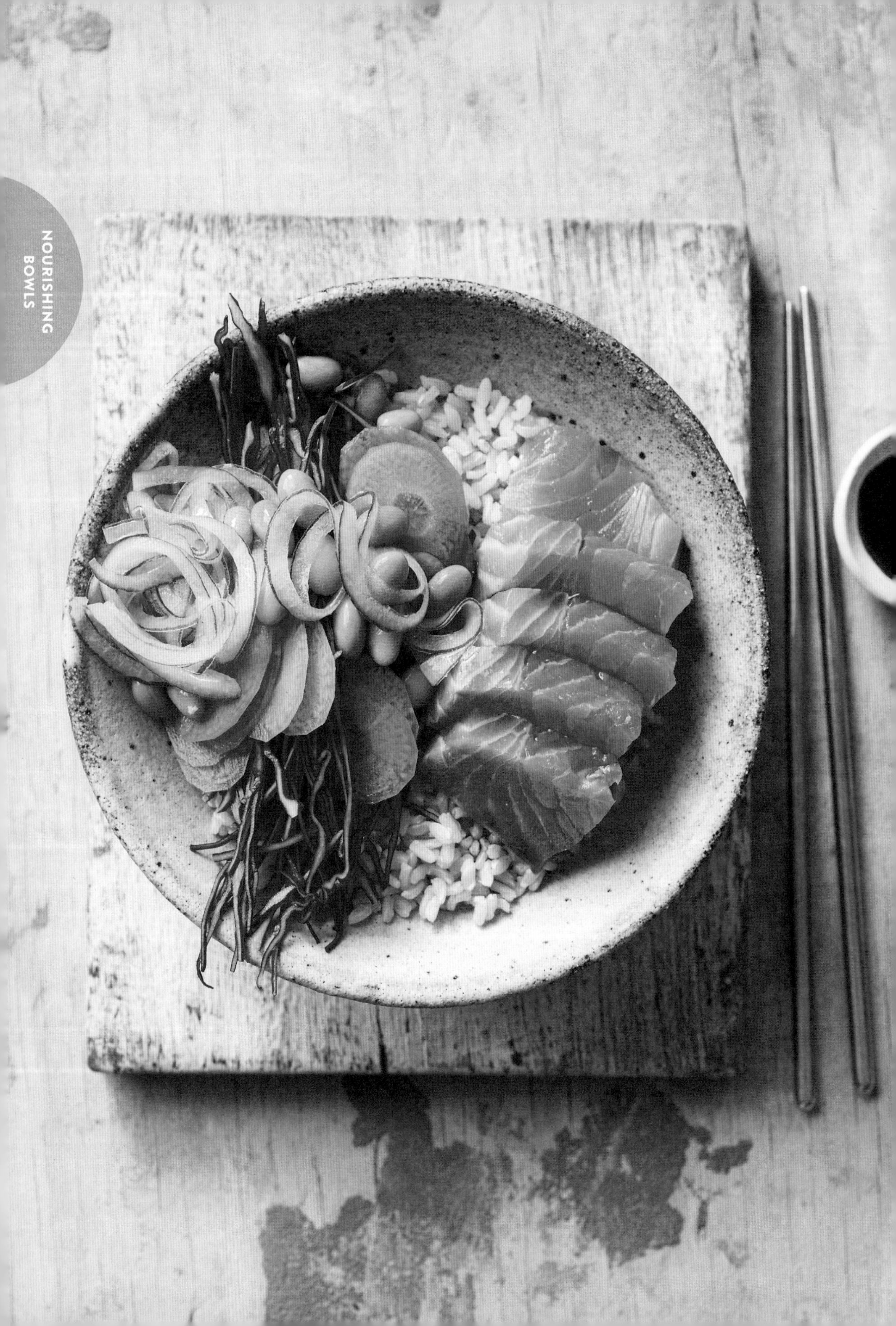

Salmon poke bowl

A poke bowl for every day of the week? These brilliant bowls are such a great way to sneak in extra vegetables and omega-3, but be careful with your dressings and toppings as they can be very high in fat and hidden sugars. If you can't find sashimi-grade salmon, buy salmon fillets and cook to your liking, or use tinned salmon. Use tamari or gluten-free soy if you're gluten intolerant.

SERVES 2 PREP TIME: **10 MINS** COOKING TIME: **25 MINS**

½ cup (100 g) brown rice, rinsed
¼ red cabbage, shredded
1 carrot, thinly sliced
1 cup (150 g) edamame beans, thawed
½ red onion, finely sliced
2 tablespoons rice wine vinegar
150 g (5½ oz) sashimi-grade salmon, thinly sliced
1 tablespoon salt-reduced soy sauce

Bring 4 cups (1 litre) of water to the boil in a saucepan. Add the rice and stir gently, then reduce the heat to a simmer and cook for 25 minutes or until tender. Drain well and spoon into two bowls.

Mix together the cabbage, carrot, edamame, onion and vinegar and spoon over the rice.

Arrange the salmon on top and drizzle with the soy sauce.

ANALYSIS SUMMARY

(PER SERVE) ENERGY 1806 KJ (429 CAL), PROTEIN 30 G, TOTAL FAT 16 G, SATURATED FAT 4 G, CARBOHYDRATE 35 G, SUGARS 20 G, DIETARY FIBRE 10 G

Chicken teriyaki poke bowl

If you've not considered eating seaweed, think again. Not only is it renowned for its iodine content, which helps regulate thyroid metabolism, but it also contains omega-3 fatty acids and antioxidants. Find it in any Asian grocery store or the Asian section of the supermarket. If you're gluten intolerant, choose gluten-free teriyaki sauce.

SERVES 2 PREP TIME: **10 MINS** COOKING TIME: **15 MINS**

1 teaspoon olive oil
300 g (10½ oz) chicken breast
125 g (4½ oz) rice stick or vermicelli noodles
1 Lebanese cucumber, shaved into ribbons
1 handful coriander (cilantro) leaves, chopped
2 tablespoons teriyaki sauce
¼ avocado, chopped
2 teaspoons sesame seeds
2 toasted nori sheets, finely sliced

Heat the oil in a frying pan over high heat. Pan-fry the chicken breast for 10–12 minutes, turning to cook all sides, until the meat is no longer pink and the juices run clear. Slice the chicken.

Place the rice noodles in a large bowl of boiling water and leave to soak for 2–3 minutes. Stir to separate the noodles, then drain well.

Mix together the noodles, cucumber, coriander and teriyaki sauce. Divide between two bowls and top with the chicken, avocado and sesame seeds. Scatter the nori over the top.

ANALYSIS SUMMARY _____

(PER SERVE) ENERGY 1666 KJ (398 CAL), PROTEIN 38 G, TOTAL FAT 10 G, SATURATED FAT 2 G, CARBOHYDRATE 37 G, SUGARS 10 G, DIETARY FIBRE 3 G

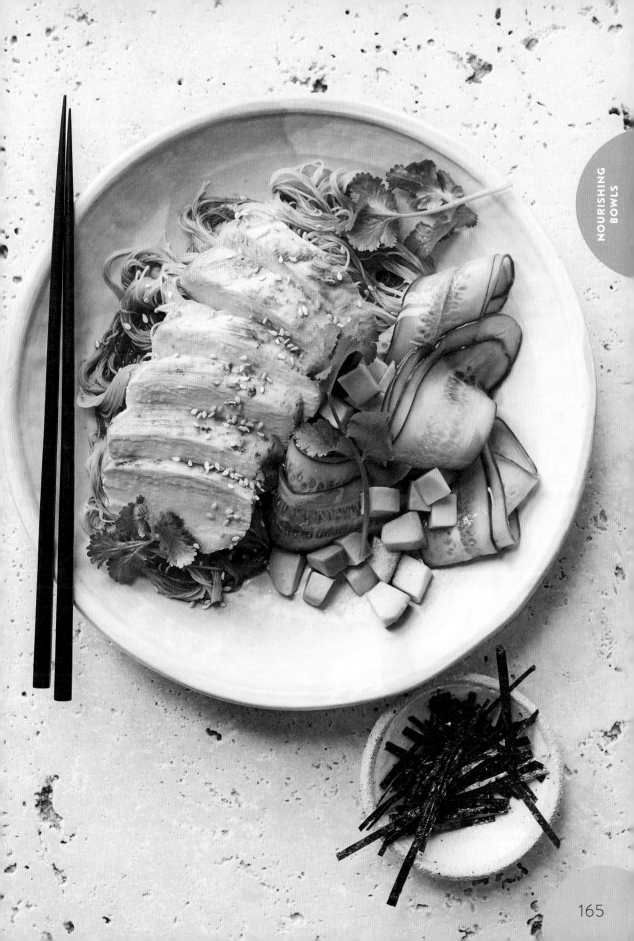

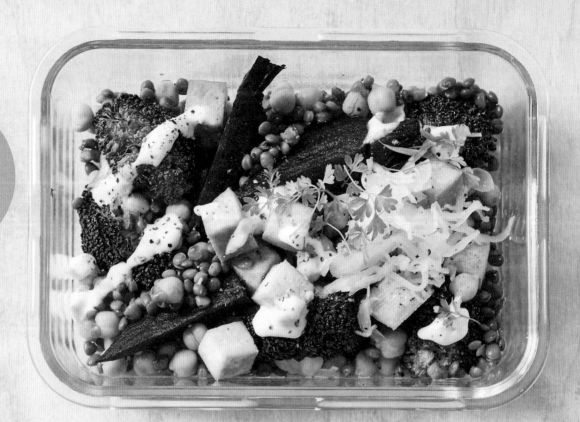
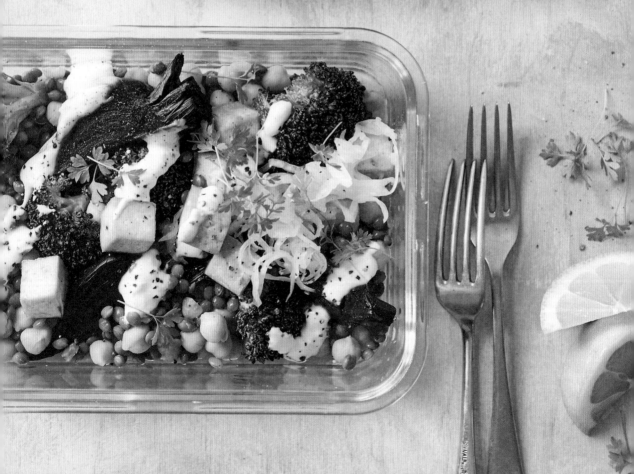

Vegetarian Buddha bowl : GF

This recipe is packed full of nutritional support for the skin. Chickpeas are low-GI and particularly high in fibre, which has been shown to help lower blood glucose levels and maintain a steady insulin response, which is less likely to trigger the hormones associated with acne. Incorporating beans is an excellent way of increasing the protein content of vegetarian meals, as well as improving your gut and bowel health. Any roast vegetables you like can be used in this. I always make extra for lunch the next day.

SERVES 2 PREP TIME: **10 MINS** COOKING TIME: **35 MINS**

1 beetroot, cut into wedges
2 teaspoons olive oil
200 g (7 oz) broccoli, chopped into florets
100 g (3½ oz) firm tofu, cubed
¾ cup (125 g) tinned brown lentils
1 cup (125 g) tinned chickpeas
3 tablespoons sauerkraut

TAHINI DRESSING
2 teaspoons tahini
2 tablespoons lemon juice
1 garlic clove, crushed
3 tablespoons low-fat Greek yoghurt

Preheat the oven to 180°C (350°F) fan-forced and line a baking tray with baking paper. Put the beetroot on the tray, coat with 1 teaspoon olive oil and season well. Roast for 20 minutes, then add the broccoli, tofu and remaining oil to the baking tray and roast for another 15 minutes.

Mix together the tahini dressing ingredients and season with salt and pepper.

Spoon the lentils, chickpeas, beetroot, broccoli and tofu into two bowls. Top with sauerkraut and drizzle with the dressing.

ANALYSIS SUMMARY

(PER SERVE) ENERGY 1654.5 KJ (396 CAL), PROTEIN 31 G, TOTAL FAT 11 G, SATURATED FAT 1 G, CARBOHYDRATE 32 G, SUGARS 7 G, DIETARY FIBRE 18 G

Smashed pumpkin with feta & pepita dukkah

Looking to impress with a simple lunch? This open sandwich has it all: it's creamy, sweet, peppery and crunchy. Pepita dukkah might sound fancy but this twist on the classic is easy to prepare and pepitas pack a punch if you are looking to boost your zinc intake. Zinc has been shown to reduce the amount of oil produced by the skin and helps heal skin damage caused by acne.

SERVES **4** PREP TIME: **10 MINS** COOKING TIME: **35 MINS**

400 g (14 oz) butternut pumpkin (squash), cut into cubes
4 eggs
4 slices rye bread or gluten-free wholegrain bread, toasted
100 g (3½ oz) reduced-fat feta cheese
1 cup (35 g) rocket (arugula)

PEPITA DUKKAH
3 tablespoons pepitas (pumpkin seeds)
2 tablespoons sesame seeds
1 teaspoon cumin seeds
1 teaspoon coriander seeds
1 teaspoon sumac

Preheat the oven to 180°C (350°F) fan-forced and line a baking tray with baking paper.

Put the pumpkin on the tray and roast for 30 minutes or until tender.

Meanwhile, to make the dukkah, toast the pepitas, sesame seeds, cumin seeds, coriander seeds and sumac in a dry frying pan over medium heat for 3 minutes or until fragrant, shaking the pan to avoid burning. Remove from the pan and grind with a spice grinder or mortar and pestle until the seeds are split but not powdery.

Meanwhile, put the eggs in a small saucepan of cold water and bring to the boil. When the water has boiled, remove from the heat and leave the eggs in the water for 2 minutes. Then run them under cold water and allow to cool slightly before peeling.

Coarsely mash the roasted pumpkin and season well.

Spread the mashed pumpkin onto warm toast, crumble the feta over the top, add a soft-boiled egg and sprinkle with dukkah. Serve with rocket.

ANALYSIS SUMMARY

(PER SERVE) ENERGY 1288 KJ (308 CAL), PROTEIN 20 G, TOTAL FAT 13 G, SATURATED FAT 4 G, CARBOHYDRATE 24 G, SUGARS 6 G, DIETARY FIBRE 6 G

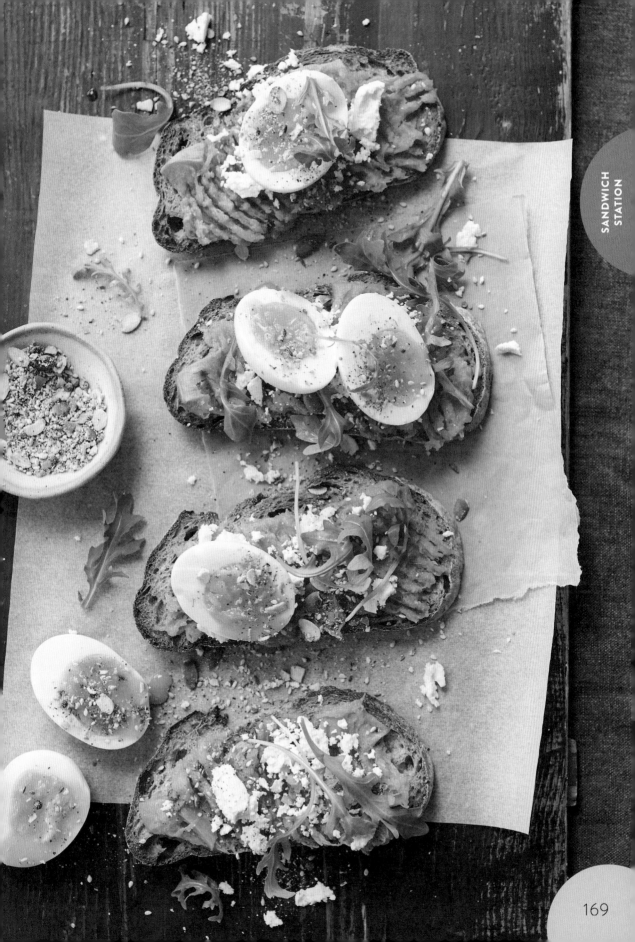

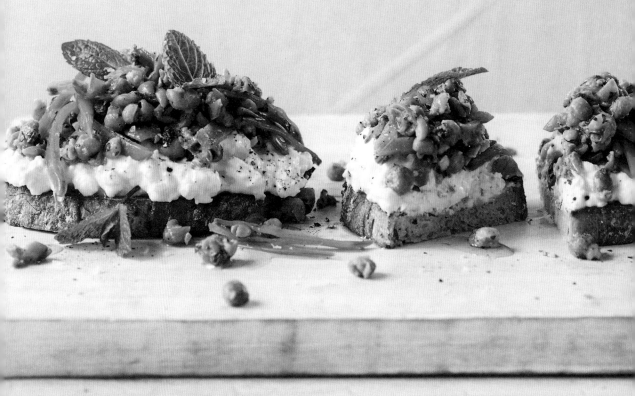

Summer pea, mint & goat's cheese tartine

The quickest tartine you have ever seen! Cottage cheese is the secret weapon in this recipe. Low in fat and high in protein and calcium, it's a perfect blank canvas for adding flavour. Peas are a great all-round vegetable: they boast low-GI carbohydrates, protein and fibre, plus vitamins and minerals, making them a staple in my diet and great food for your skin.

SERVES **2** PREP TIME: **10 MINS** COOKING TIME: **5 MINS**

200 g (7 oz) reduced-fat cottage cheese
50 g (1¾ oz) goat's cheese
200 g (7 oz) peas
juice of 1 lemon
1 tablespoon dijon mustard
1 garlic clove, crushed
1 tablespoon extra virgin olive oil
1 teaspoon cajun spice
½ bunch mint, leaves chopped
200 g (7 oz) snow peas, sliced diagonally
2 slices sourdough bread or gluten-free wholegrain
   bread, toasted

Mix together the cottage cheese and goat's cheese.

Coarsely mash together the peas, lemon juice, mustard, garlic, oil, cajun spice and most of the mint. Season with salt and pepper, then stir in the snow peas.

To assemble, spread the cheese mixture on the toast and top with the pea mixture and remaining mint.

ANALYSIS SUMMARY ⎯⎯⎯⎯⎯⎯⎯⎯⎯⎯⎯⎯⎯⎯⎯⎯⎯⎯⎯⎯⎯⎯⎯⎯⎯⎯⎯⎯

(PER SERVE) ENERGY 1693 KJ (405 CAL), PROTEIN 32 G, TOTAL FAT 10 G, SATURATED FAT 6 G, CARBOHYDRATE 37 G, SUGARS 14 G, DIETARY FIBRE 12 G

Lamb wraps with tzatziki

This is an easy lunch idea for when you have leftover roast lamb – a great source of iron. Tzatziki is a perfect substitute for creamy dressings that can be loaded with saturated fat. Yoghurt is also high in calcium and zinc, which has been shown to be beneficial for acne and rosacea. This sauce can be made in bulk and stored in the fridge for 1 week.

SERVES **4** PREP TIME: **10 MINS** COOKING TIME: **20 MINS**

1 eggplant (aubergine), sliced into thin rounds
2 teaspoons olive oil
400 g (14 oz) lean lamb fillet
4 wholemeal flatbreads or gluten-free wraps
½ cos lettuce, shredded
½ red onion, finely sliced

TZATZIKI
½ cup (130 g) low-fat Greek yoghurt
½ Lebanese cucumber, finely chopped
juice of ½ lemon
½ garlic clove, crushed

Heat a chargrill pan over medium heat. Arrange the eggplant slices in a single layer, brush with oil and season with salt and pepper. Cook, turning occasionally, for 10 minutes, until the eggplant is tender, then remove from the pan.

Add the lamb to the pan and season with salt and pepper. Cook for 5 minutes on each side or until medium–rare. Rest for 5 minutes, then cut into slices.

To make the tzatziki, combine all the ingredients in a small bowl.

Put the lettuce, eggplant, onion and lamb into the bread. Drizzle with the tzatziki and fold up the bread. Serve toasted or as is.

ANALYSIS SUMMARY

(PER SERVE) ENERGY 1686 KJ (403 CAL), PROTEIN 38 G, TOTAL FAT 8 G, SATURATED FAT 3 G, CARBOHYDRATE 39 G, SUGARS 10 G, DIETARY FIBRE 9 G

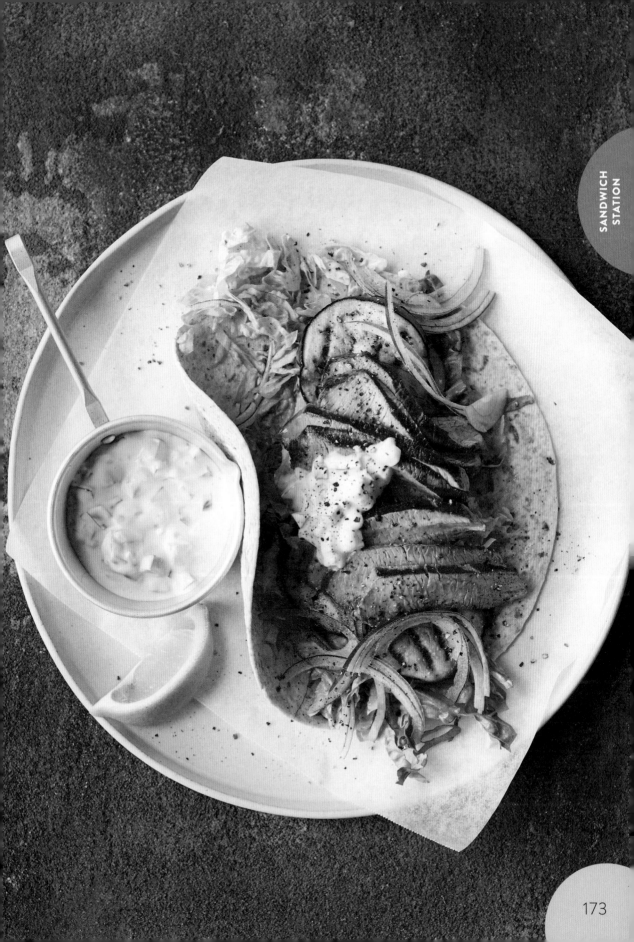

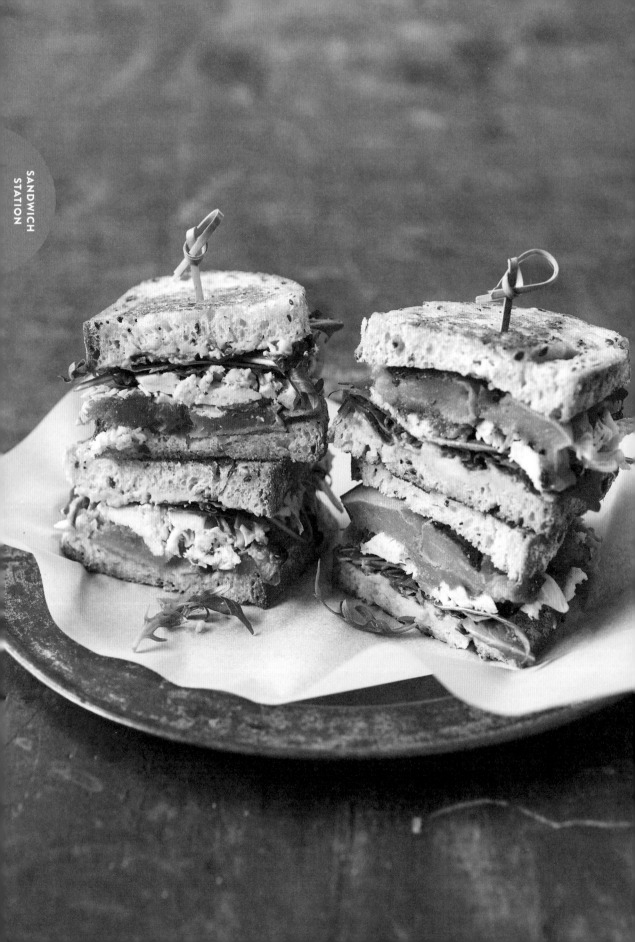

Leftover roast chicken dinner toastie

This recipe is another perfect idea for using leftovers from the night before. Substitute any lean meat and roasted root vegetables you have in the fridge and it's a complete meal on the go!

SERVES 2 PREP TIME: 5 MINS COOKING TIME: 5 MINS

200 g (7 oz) roast pumpkin (squash) or other veg, mashed
4 slices wholegrain sourdough or gluten-free wholegrain bread
½ avocado
200 g (7 oz) roast chicken or other lean meat, shredded
1 cup (35 g) rocket (arugula)

Spread the pumpkin over 2 slices of bread, and the avocado over the other slices.

Top the pumpkin with chicken and rocket, and place the avocado bread on top to make a sandwich. Toast in a sandwich press for 5 minutes or until golden.

ANALYSIS SUMMARY _____

(PER SERVE) ENERGY 1761 KJ (421 CAL), PROTEIN 40 G, TOTAL FAT 11 G, SATURATED FAT 3 G, CARBOHYDRATE 37 G, SUGARS 8 G, DIETARY FIBRE 6 G

Roast beef roll with beetroot & horseradish cream

This recipe takes roast beef rolls to another level. I could tell you it's high in iron for wound healing and antioxidants for immune function, but that's not why you'll keep coming back for more. Try roast beef with sweet earthy beetroot and the zesty heat of horseradish cream and you'll be hooked. Choose a good-quality tinned beetroot with minimal sugar for this.

SERVES 2 PREP TIME: **5 MINS** COOKING TIME: **5 MINS**

1 tablespoon reduced-fat crème fraiche
2 teaspoons horseradish
2 wholemeal or gluten-free bread rolls, cut in half
1 cup (35 g) rocket (arugula)
6 slices good-quality tinned beetroot
150 g (5½ oz) roast beef, sliced
¼ red onion, finely sliced

Mix together the crème fraiche and horseradish. Spread over the bottom half of the bread rolls.

Add the rocket, beetroot and roast beef, then scatter with the onion.

Put the tops on the rolls and toast in a sandwich press for 5 minutes or until golden.

ANALYSIS SUMMARY

(PER SERVE) ENERGY 1578 KJ (377 CAL), PROTEIN 34 G, TOTAL FAT 9 G, SATURATED FAT 2 G, CARBOHYDRATE 38 G, SUGARS 8 G, DIETARY FIBRE 7 G

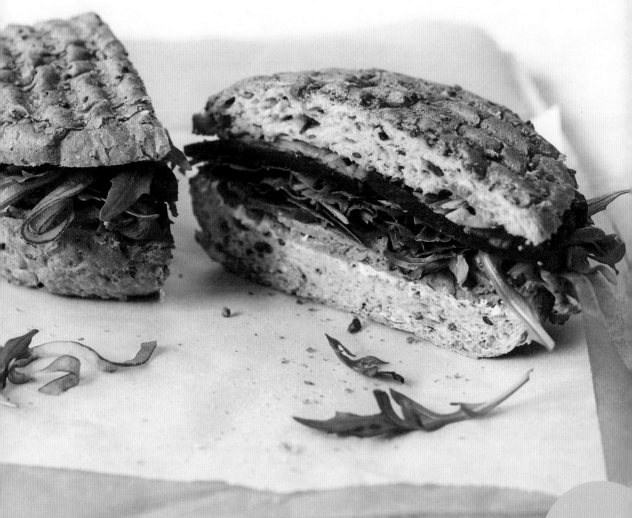

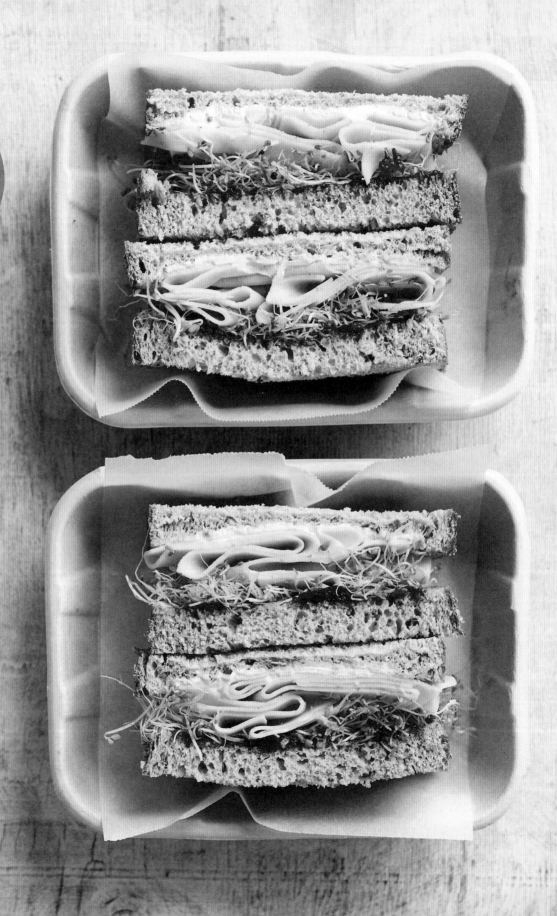

Turkey, cranberry, cream cheese & alfalfa sandwich

Rye bread is high in fibre, plus its GI is lower than many other products made from wheat. This makes rye a great choice for a healthy digestive system, which promotes clearer, brighter-looking skin.

SERVES **2** PREP TIME: **5 MINS**

4 slices rye bread or gluten-free wholegrain bread
1 tablespoon reduced-fat cream cheese
200 g (7 oz) turkey breast, sliced
½ cup (30 g) alfalfa sprouts
1 tablespoon good-quality cranberry sauce

Spread 2 slices of rye bread with cream cheese. Top with the turkey breast and alfalfa sprouts.

Spread the cranberry sauce onto the other 2 slices of rye bread and lay on top to make sandwiches.

ANALYSIS SUMMARY

(PER SERVE) ENERGY 1623 KJ (388 CAL), PROTEIN 37 G, TOTAL FAT 8 G, SATURATED FAT 3 G, CARBOHYDRATE 37 G, SUGARS 7 G, DIETARY FIBRE 6 G

The Reuben on rye

With its perfectly balanced big flavours, the Reuben is the king of deli sandwiches for a reason. All I've done here is make it healthier for you. Corned beef is traditionally preserved with high amounts of salt, but by choosing salt-reduced options you can reduce the sodium load in this sandwich.

SERVES **2** PREP TIME: **5 MINS** COOKING TIME: **5 MINS**

1 tablespoon dijon mustard
4 slices rye bread or gluten-free wholegrain bread
200 g (7 oz) lean salt-reduced corned beef, sliced
½ cup (75 g) sauerkraut
40 g (1½ oz) reduced-fat cheddar cheese, sliced

Spread the mustard over 2 slices of rye bread. Place corned beef on top of each slice, along with the sauerkraut and cheddar.

Top with another slice of rye bread and toast in a sandwich press for 5 minutes or until the cheese is melted.

ANALYSIS SUMMARY

(PER SERVE) ENERGY 1592 KJ (381 CAL), PROTEIN 30 G, TOTAL FAT 10 G, SATURATED FAT 4 G, CARBOHYDRATE 36 G, SUGARS 3 G, DIETARY FIBRE 9 G

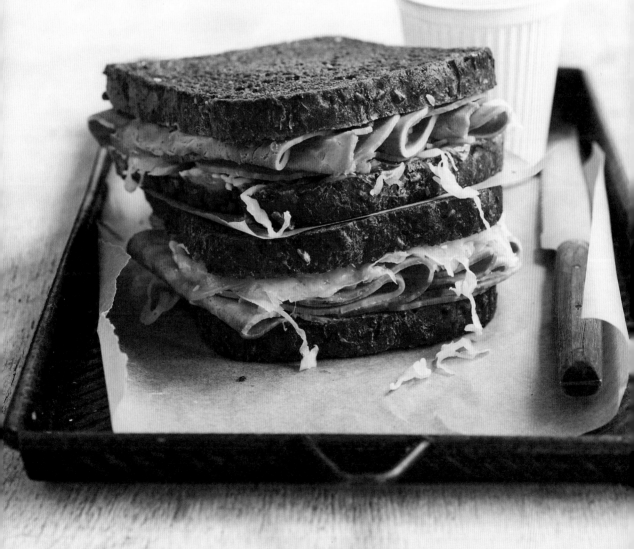

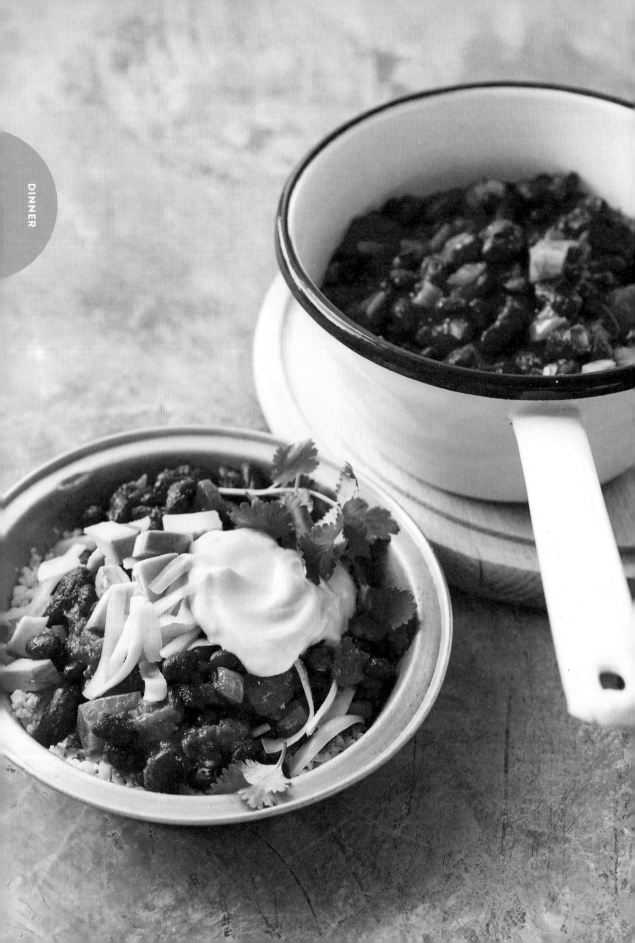

Black bean chilli with cauliflower rice : GF

Snuggle up with a steaming bowl of this chilli with all its glorious toppings. Even devoted meat-eaters will be satisfied. Black beans and kidney beans bump up the protein, fibre and iron content, which are important for gut health and cell renewal.

SERVES **4** PREP TIME: **10 MINS** COOKING TIME: **35 MINS**

1 cauliflower, chopped into florets
1 teaspoon olive oil
1 onion, chopped
2 zucchini (courgettes), grated
2 tablespoons Mexican spice mix
400 g (14 oz) tinned black beans, rinsed
400 g (14 oz) tinned kidney beans, rinsed

400 g (14 oz) tinned chopped tomatoes
½ cup (50 g) grated reduced-fat cheddar cheese
½ small avocado
¾ cup (200 g) low-fat Greek yoghurt
½ bunch coriander (cilantro)

Preheat the oven to 180°C (350°F) fan-forced.

To make the cauliflower rice, put the cauliflower on a baking tray and season with salt and pepper. Bake for 20 minutes or until tender and starting to brown. Transfer to a food processor and process until it resembles rice. Cover and set aside.

Heat the oil in a frying pan over medium–high heat. Add the onion and sauté, stirring, for 3 minutes or until soft. Add the zucchini and cook for a further 2 minutes. Add the Mexican spice mix and cook for 1 minute or until fragrant. Add the black beans, kidney beans and tomatoes. Reduce the heat to low–medium and simmer for 10 minutes or until thickened slightly.

Serve the chilli over the cauliflower rice. Top with cheese, avocado and yoghurt and garnish with coriander leaves.

ANALYSIS SUMMARY

(PER SERVE) ENERGY 1472 KJ (352 CAL), PROTEIN 23 G, TOTAL FAT 9 G, SATURATED FAT 3 G, CARBOHYDRATE 38 G, SUGARS 14 G, DIETARY FIBRE 17 G

Lentil shepherd's pie with cheesy cauliflower crust

Another great alternative for a non-meat day. Lentils are rich in protein, low-GI carb and fibre. But the most exciting part of this dish is the cheesy cauliflower crust that you'll just want to break into. Don't despair if you don't eat dairy – you can replace cottage cheese with silken tofu. If you're gluten intolerant, look for a gluten-free worcestershire sauce.

SERVES 4 PREP TIME: **20 MINS** COOKING TIME: **55 MINS**

1 tablespoon olive oil
1 onion, chopped
1 carrot, chopped
2 x 400 g (14 oz) tins brown lentils,
   drained and rinsed
2 cups (500 ml) salt-reduced
   vegetable stock
1 tablespoon worcestershire sauce

1 teaspoon dried rosemary
1 cup (140 g) frozen peas

CRUST
500 g (1 lb 2 oz) cauliflower florets
400 g (14 oz) reduced-fat cottage cheese
1 tablespoon dijon mustard

Preheat the oven to 180°C (350°F) fan-forced.

Heat the oil in a frying pan over medium–high heat. Add the onion and sauté for 3 minutes or until translucent. Add the carrot, lentils, stock, worcestershire sauce and rosemary.

Reduce the heat to low, cover and simmer for 15 minutes or until the stock begins to reduce. Crush some of the lentils with a wooden spoon to thicken. Add the peas and season, then remove from the heat. Transfer to a large baking dish, or individual dishes.

To make the crust, steam the cauliflower in the microwave or over a saucepan of simmering water for 5–10 minutes until tender. Add the cottage cheese and mustard, then season with salt and pepper and mash until creamy. Spread evenly over the lentil mixture.

Bake for about 25 minutes until golden brown.

ANALYSIS SUMMARY

(PER SERVE) ENERGY 1459 KJ (349 CAL), PROTEIN 28 G, TOTAL FAT 7 G, SATURATED FAT 2 G, CARBOHYDRATE 35 G, SUGARS 16 G, DIETARY FIBRE 13 G

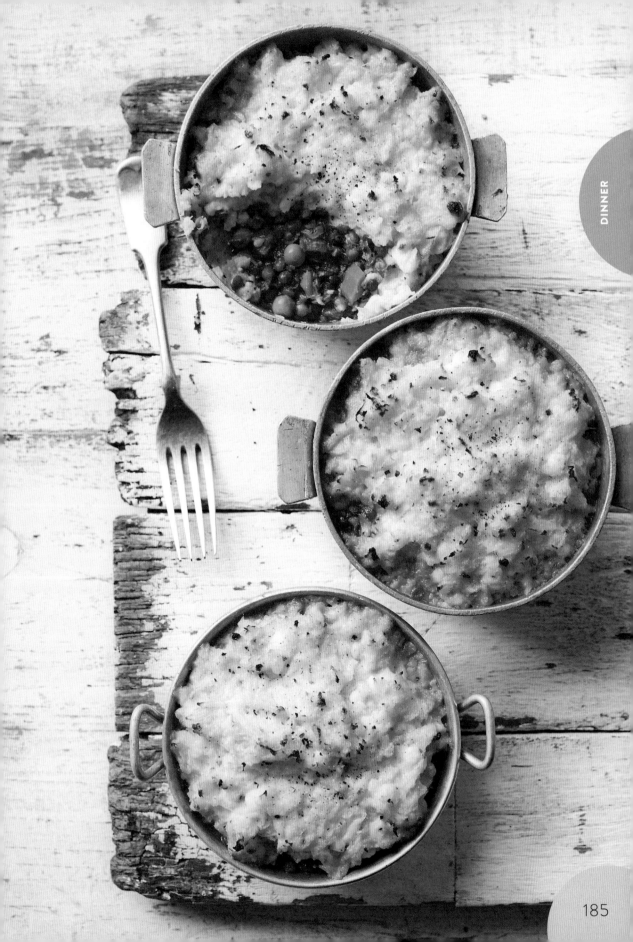

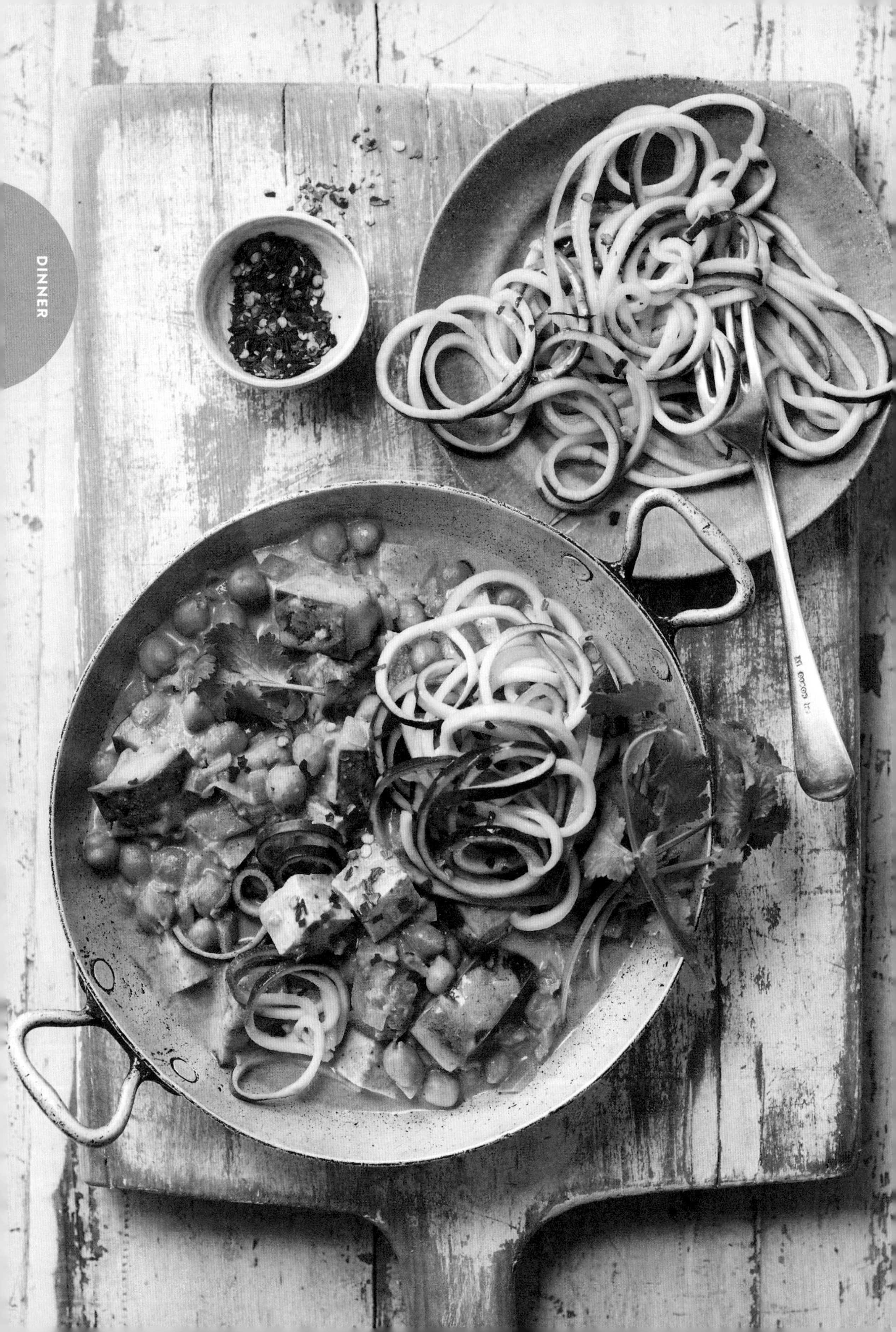

Tofu & eggplant curry with zoodles : GF

It's important to have a balance of protein and carbohydrate when eating vegetarian; it can be a real challenge to include enough protein. Tofu is a great plant-based source of protein, plus it's rich in isoflavones, which can help protect against age-related disease. Using zucchini noodles is a delicious way to keep the carbohydrate down while increasing fibre. If you don't have the spices on hand, use ready-made yellow curry paste, but be aware that it can contain preservatives.

SERVES 4 PREP TIME: **20 MINS** COOKING TIME: **25 MINS**

4 zucchini (courgettes)
1 tablespoon olive oil
1 onion, chopped
2 garlic cloves, crushed
2 teaspoons grated fresh ginger
2 tablespoons garam masala
2 teaspoons ground cumin
2 teaspoons dried chilli flakes

1 teaspoon ground turmeric
1 cup (250 ml) light coconut milk
2 cups (500 ml) salt-reduced vegetable stock
1 eggplant (aubergine), cut into cubes
400 g (14 oz) tin chickpeas, drained
400 g (14 oz) firm tofu, cubed
1 bunch coriander (cilantro)

To make the zucchini noodles, shave each zucchini with a hand spiraliser, a mandoline or a vegetable peeler to resemble noodles.

Heat the oil in a large saucepan over medium–high heat. Add the onion and sauté for 2–3 minutes until it softens. Add the garlic, ginger, garam masala, cumin, chilli flakes and turmeric and toast for 1 minute, stirring constantly.

Add the coconut milk and stock and bring to a simmer. Add the eggplant and cook for 10 minutes or until it is soft but not mushy.

Stir the chickpeas and tofu into the curry and let them heat through for another 5–10 minutes.

Toss the zucchini noodles in a hot wok for a couple of minutes to soften them slightly.

Serve the curry with zoodles, and scatter coriander over the top.

ANALYSIS SUMMARY

(PER SERVE) ENERGY 1503 KJ (360 CAL), PROTEIN 26 G, TOTAL FAT 13 G, SATURATED FAT 3 G, CARBOHYDRATE 27 G, SUGARS 16 G, DIETARY FIBRE 14 G

Korean beef bibimbap

Not all bibimbaps are created equal. Some commercial versions can contain a whopping 130 grams of carbohydrate in just one serve! This version uses brown rice, with a lower GI, with lean protein and vegetables for a dinner that won't leave you feeling sluggish. Use tamari or gluten-free soy if you're gluten intolerant.

SERVES 4 PREP TIME: **10 MINS** COOKING TIME: **40 MINS**

1 garlic clove, crushed
2 teaspoons grated fresh ginger
2 tablespoons soy sauce
350 g (12 oz) lean beef stir-fry strips
¾ cup (150 g) brown rice
1 tablespoon sesame oil

4 eggs
2 carrots, shaved into ribbons
2 Lebanese cucumbers,
  cut into matchsticks
2 cups (230 g) bean sprouts
2 teaspoons sesame seeds

Mix together the garlic, ginger and soy sauce. Pour half into a large bowl, add the beef strips and set aside to marinate.

Bring 400 ml (14 fl oz) water to the boil in a saucepan. Add the rice, stir, then cover and reduce the heat to low. Simmer for 25 minutes, then remove from the heat and keep covered for another 5 minutes, or until the rice is tender and all the water has been absorbed.

Heat the sesame oil in a frying pan over medium–high heat. Add half the marinated beef strips to the pan and cook for 1–2 minutes until cooked through. Transfer to a bowl and cook the rest of the beef.

Return the pan to medium–high heat. Crack in the eggs and fry for 4–5 minutes.

Spoon the rice into four bowls, add the beef strips, carrot, cucumber and bean sprouts and top with an egg. Drizzle with the remaining soy mixture and sprinkle with sesame seeds.

ANALYSIS SUMMARY ⎯⎯⎯⎯⎯⎯⎯⎯⎯⎯⎯⎯⎯⎯⎯⎯⎯

(PER SERVE) ENERGY 1651 KJ (394 CAL), PROTEIN 35 G, TOTAL FAT 10 G, SATURATED FAT 2 G, CARBOHYDRATE 38 G, SUGARS 7 G, DIETARY FIBRE 5 G

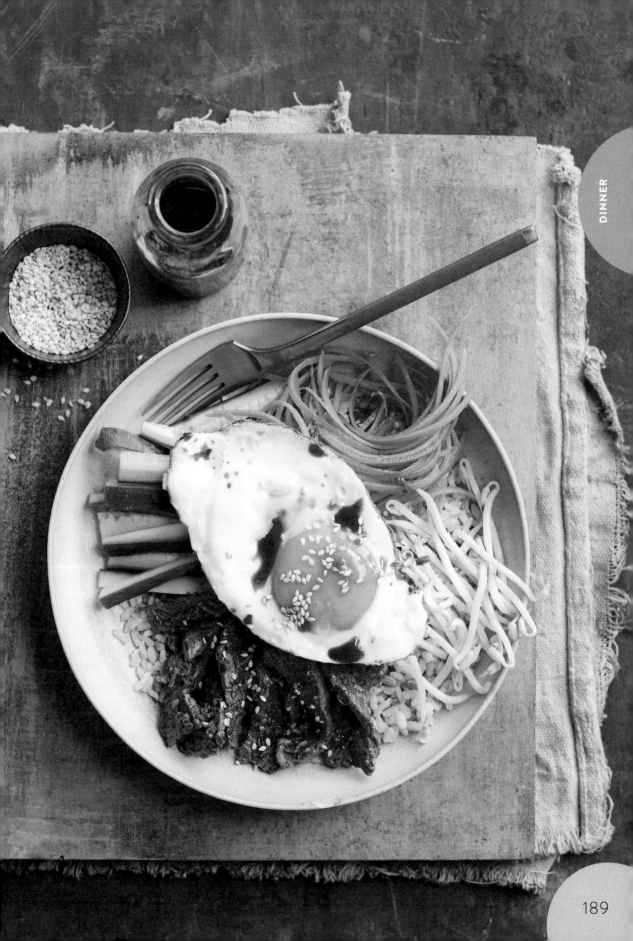

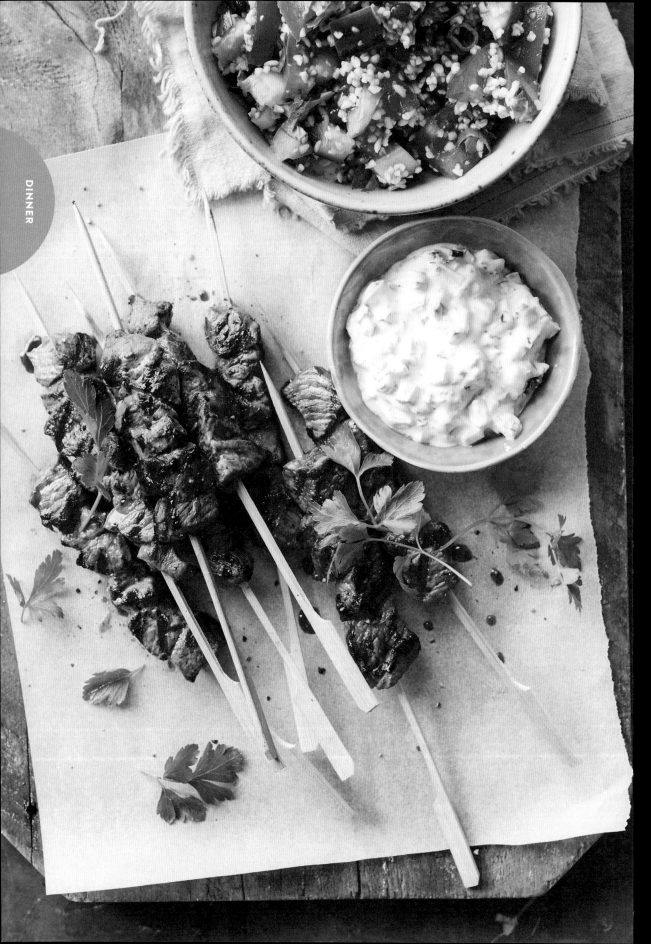

Lamb skewers with pomegranate tabbouleh & mint & cucumber yoghurt

Yes, I said pomegranate tabbouleh! You need to try this. I love bulgur wheat, a wholewheat grain that is high fibre and low GI. If you are gluten intolerant, try replacing it with quinoa.

SERVES **4** PREP TIME: **20 MINS** COOKING TIME: **30 MINS**

¾ cup (130 g) bulgur wheat
1 tablespoon olive oil
3 tablespoons lemon juice
3 tomatoes, chopped
2 Lebanese cucumbers, chopped
1 large handful mint, chopped
1 large handful flat-leaf parsley, chopped
2 spring onions (scallions), finely chopped
juice and seeds of 1 pomegranate
500 g (1 lb 2 oz) lamb fillet, diced

MINT AND CUCUMBER YOGHURT
½ cup (130 g) low-fat Greek yoghurt
1 Lebanese cucumber, finely chopped
2 tablespoons finely chopped mint
½ garlic clove, crushed

To make the mint and cucumber yoghurt, combine all the ingredients.

To make the tabbouleh, put the bulgur wheat in a bowl, add 1½ cups (375 ml) of boiling water and leave for 20 minutes. Drain any excess water and stir in the oil, lemon juice, tomato, cucumber, mint, parsley, spring onions and pomegranate seeds and juice. Cover and refrigerate while you prepare the lamb.

Heat a frying pan over high heat. Thread the lamb onto skewers and season with salt and pepper. Cook the kebabs for 10–12 minutes, turning regularly to brown on all sides. Serve with the tabbouleh and a dollop of mint and cucumber yoghurt.

ANALYSIS SUMMARY _____

(PER SERVE) ENERGY 1713 KJ (410 CAL) , PROTEIN 34 G , TOTAL FAT 11 G, SATURATED FAT 3 G, CARBOHYDRATE 36 G, SUGARS 16 G , DIETARY FIBRE 12 G

Corned beef with roasted brussels sprouts & pear quinoa : GF

This is the perfect winter meal – completely comforting and nourishing when your body needs it most. I've given these old-fashioned ingredients a new twist. Always choose lean, salt-reduced corned beef to minimise saturated fat and sodium. Leftover corned beef can be used in breakfast hash and lunch sandwiches, so feel free to cook extra. Look for a good-quality onion relish with minimal sugar.

SERVES **4** PREP TIME: **10 MINS** COOKING TIME: **1 HR**

300 g (10½ oz) lean, salt-reduced corned
  beef (silverside)
1 onion, chopped
500 g (1 lb 2 oz) brussels sprouts, halved
3 pears, quartered
1 tablespoon olive oil
3 tablespoons slivered almonds

1 cup (200 g) quinoa
½ cup (75 g) sauerkraut
½ bunch chives, chopped
2 tablespoons red wine vinegar
3 tablespoons dijon mustard
2 tablespoons good-quality onion relish

Place the corned beef and onion in a large saucepan with enough water to cover. Cover with a lid and simmer over low–medium heat for 1 hour or until the meat is tender. Preheat the oven to 180°C (350°F) fan-forced and line a large baking tray with baking paper.

Steam the sprouts over a pan of simmering water for 10 minutes, or microwave for 5 minutes, until slightly softened.

Put the sprouts in a bowl with the pears and toss with the oil, salt and pepper. Arrange in a single layer on the baking tray and roast for 15 minutes or until tender and starting to colour. Sprinkle with slivered almonds and roast for another 5 minutes.

Rinse the quinoa and put it in a saucepan with 2 cups (500 ml) water. Bring to the boil, then reduce the heat to medium, cover and cook for 15 minutes or until tender. Add the sprouts, pears, sauerkraut and chives to the quinoa.

Mix the vinegar, 2 tablespoons of the mustard and the onion relish and pour over the quinoa. Toss to coat. Serve the pear quinoa topped with shredded corned beef and the remaining mustard.

ANALYSIS SUMMARY

(PER SERVE) ENERGY 1884 KJ (450 CAL), PROTEIN 35 G, TOTAL FAT 13 G, SATURATED FAT 2 G, CARBOHYDRATE 37 G, SUGARS 24 G, DIETARY FIBRE 16 G

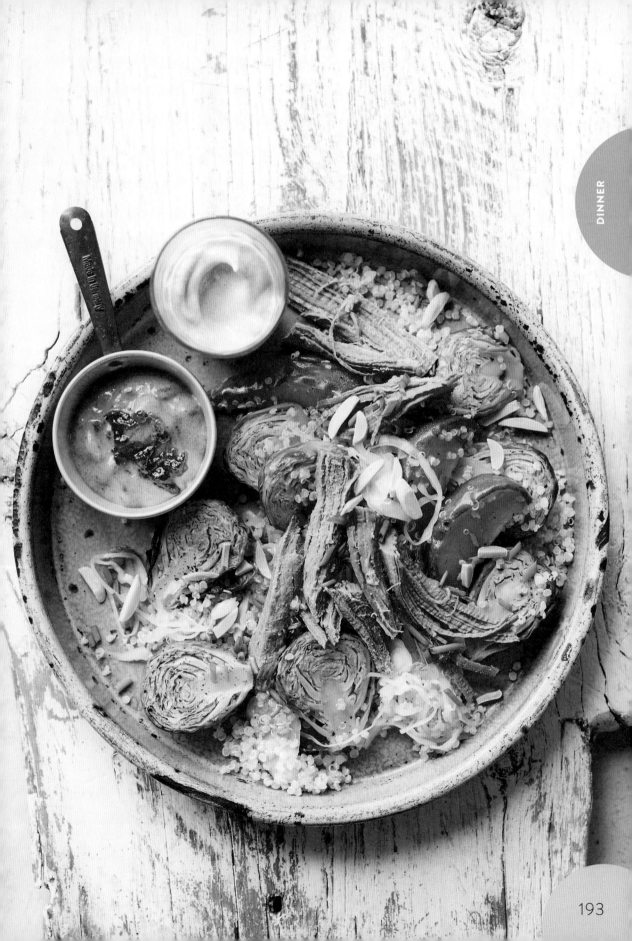

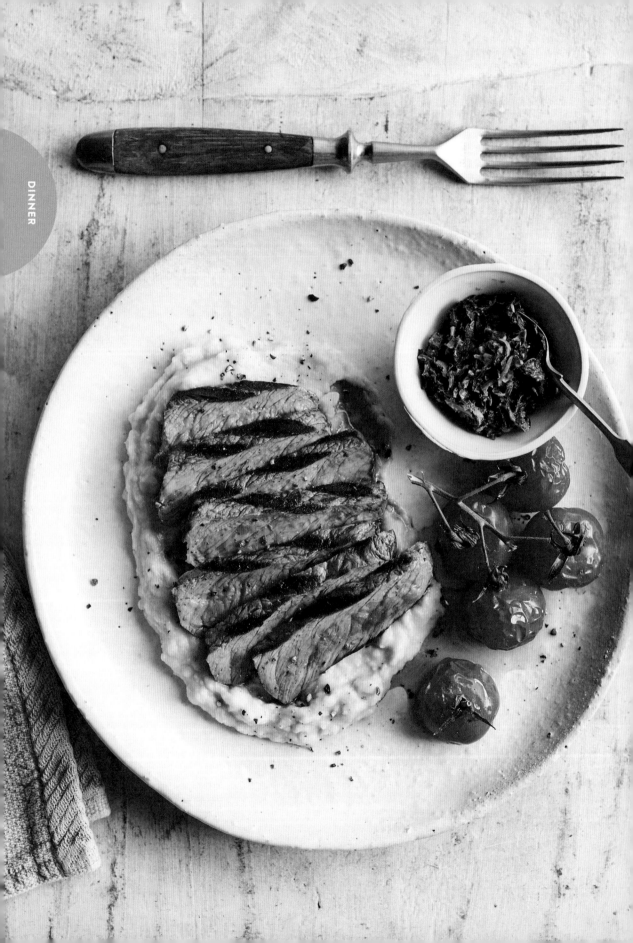

Steak with salsa verde & white beans : GF

This recipe is so simple and so good: high in iron for cell rejuvenation, prebiotics for gut health and low-GI carbohydrates for steady blood sugar levels. The herbaceous zestiness of the salsa verde lifts this meal to new heights and it can be used in so many ways. Ready-made versions often contain a lot of oil, so why not try making your own?

SERVES 2 PREP TIME: **15 MINS** COOKING TIME: **10 MINS**

200 g (7 oz) fillet steak
8 cherry tomatoes on the vine
400 g (14 oz) tin cannellini beans,
 drained and rinsed
3 tablespoons milk

SALSA VERDE
1 handful basil, finely chopped
1 handful flat-leaf parsley, finely chopped
1 tablespoon capers, rinsed
1 tablespoon olive oil
2 tablespoons white wine vinegar
1 tablespoon dijon mustard
½ garlic clove, crushed

To make the salsa verde, blitz all the ingredients in a blender until just combined but not smooth.

Preheat a chargrill pan over medium–high heat. Put the steak and cherry tomatoes in the pan and season with salt and pepper. Grill for 6–8 minutes, turning the steak once, for medium–rare. Rest the steak for 5 minutes, then slice.

Meanwhile, put the cannellini beans and milk in a small saucepan and season with salt and pepper. Bring to a simmer, then remove from the heat and blend to a purée.

To serve, spoon the bean purée onto two plates and top with steak. Serve with cherry tomatoes and salsa verde.

ANALYSIS SUMMARY _____

(PER SERVE) ENERGY 1886 KJ (451 CAL), PROTEIN 36 G, TOTAL FAT 17 G, SATURATED FAT 4 G, CARBOHYDRATE 26 G, SUGARS 6 G, DIETARY FIBRE 16 G

Crispy fish tacos : GF

Fish tacos are the hottest thing around right now. The problem is that the ones in restaurants are usually deep-fried and covered in mayonnaise, making them not nearly as healthy as they could be. This recipe has everything you love about fresh Mexican flavours and crispy fish, without the added inches on your waistline.

SERVES 4 PREP TIME: **20 MINS** COOKING TIME: **20 MINS**

500 g (1 lb 2 oz) firm white fish,
    cut into thick strips
3 tablespoons polenta
2 teaspoons olive oil
4 mini corn tortillas
¼ red cabbage, shredded
1 small avocado, diced
lime wedges, to serve

SALSA
4 tomatoes, diced
1 Lebanese cucumber, diced
½ red onion, finely diced
1 handful coriander (cilantro), chopped
1 small red chilli, seeded and finely chopped
juice of 1 lime

To make the salsa, mix together all the ingredients and season with salt and pepper.

Toss the fish in polenta and salt and pepper to coat.

Heat the oil in a large non-stick frying pan over medium heat. Cook the fish, in batches, for 2 minutes on each side or until crisp and just cooked through. Drain on paper towel.

Meanwhile, lightly toast the tortillas in a dry frying pan.

Fill the tortillas with cabbage, salsa and fish. Top with avocado and a squeeze of lime.

ANALYSIS SUMMARY _____

(PER SERVE) ENERGY 2016 KJ (482 CAL), PROTEIN 35 G, TOTAL FAT 14 G, SATURATED FAT 3 G, CARBOHYDRATE 49 G, SUGARS 8 G, DIETARY FIBRE 8 G

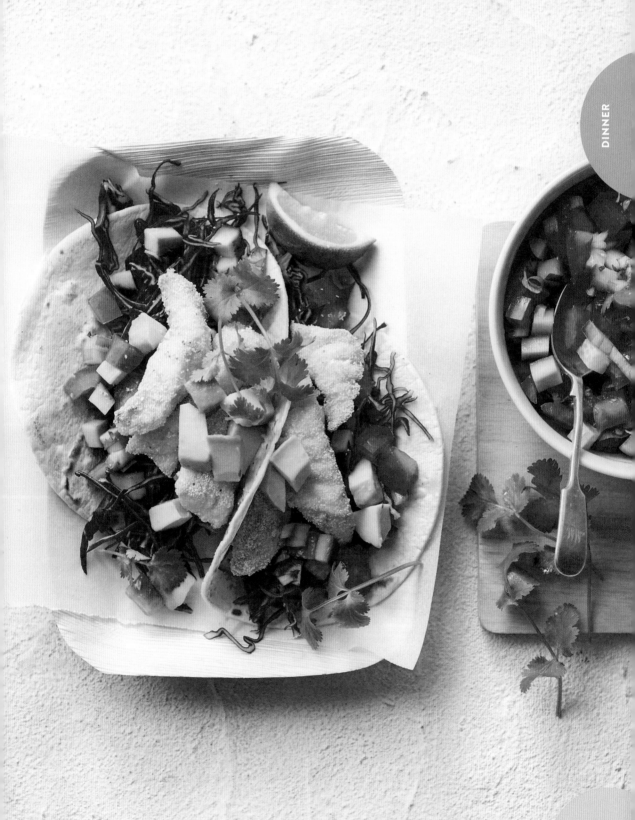

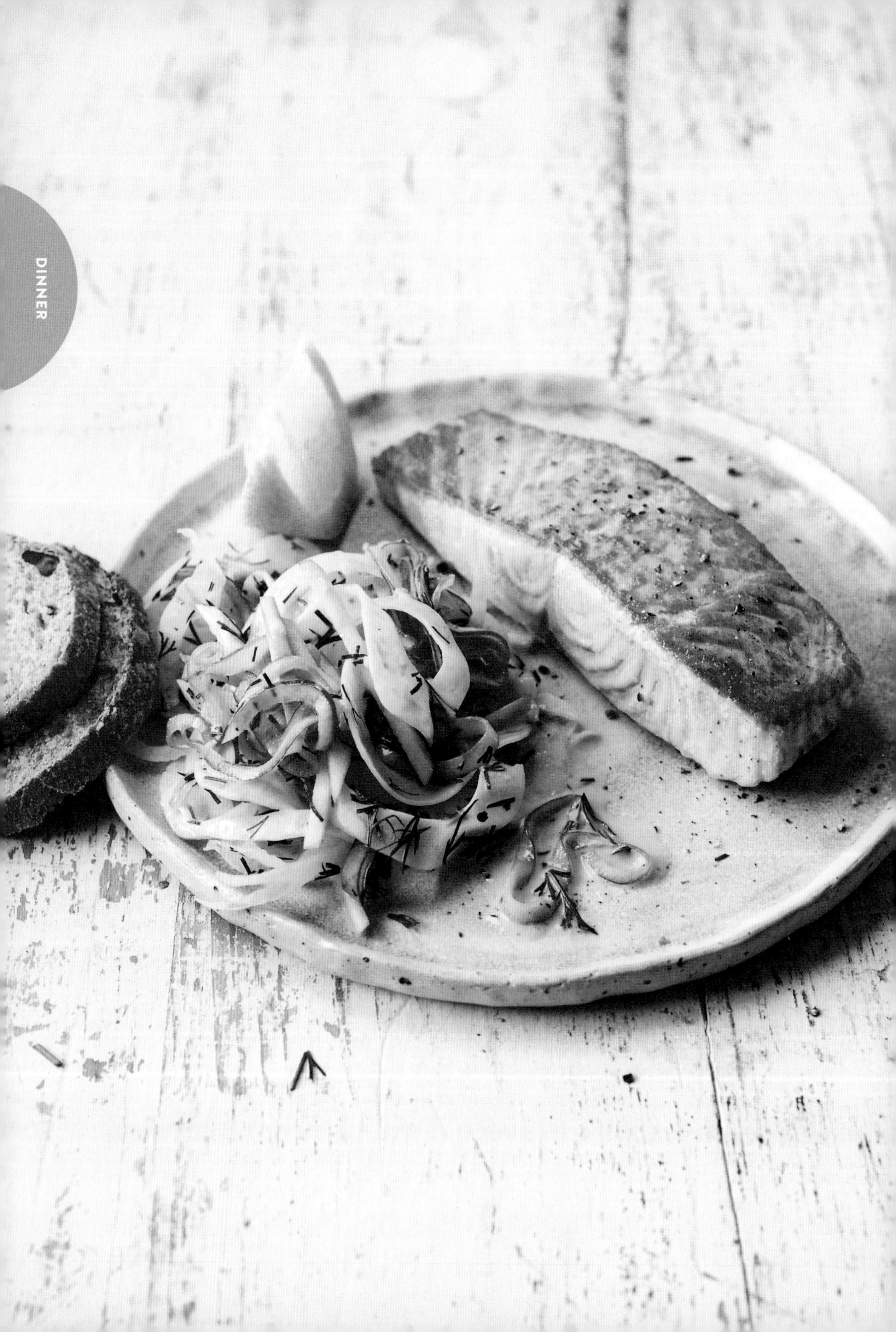

Grilled salmon with apple slaw & pickled onions : GF

This recipe is one of my all-time favourites for good reason. High in omega-3, protein and fibre, it's a no-brainer for your body but so ridiculously delicious you won't even notice it's super-healthy! Traditional coleslaws can be high in saturated fat, so using yoghurt and horseradish is a smart way to add creaminess and zing without the calories. You'll need to make the pickled onion at least 1 hour before serving.

SERVES 2 PREP TIME: **1 HR** COOKING TIME: **10 MINS**

1 fennel bulb, tough outer layer removed, finely shredded
1 granny smith apple, thinly sliced
½ bunch dill, chopped
3 tablespoons low-fat Greek yoghurt
juice of 1 lemon
2 teaspoons horseradish cream
1 tablespoon olive oil

300 g (10½ oz) salmon fillets
gluten-free bread, to serve

PICKLED ONION
3 tablespoons red wine vinegar
2 teaspoons honey
½ red onion, finely sliced

To make the pickled onion, whisk together the vinegar, honey and a pinch of salt in a small bowl, then add the onion, making sure that it is fully submerged in the liquid. Set aside for at least an hour until softened, then drain, reserving the pickling liquid.

Toss together the fennel, apple, dill and pickled onion. Whisk together the pickling liquid, yoghurt, lemon juice and the horseradish cream to make a dressing, then toss through the slaw.

Heat the oil in a frying pan over high heat. Season the salmon with salt and pepper and cook, skin-side down, for 4 minutes until the skin is crisp. Turn and cook for a further 2 minutes until golden.

Serve the salmon with apple slaw and gluten-free bread.

ANALYSIS SUMMARY

(PER SERVE) ENERGY 2297 KJ (550 CAL), PROTEIN 40 G, TOTAL FAT 22 G, SATURATED FAT 5 G, CARBOHYDRATE 40 G, SUGARS 22 G, DIETARY FIBRE 8 G

Dukkah roast chicken with root vegetable crumble

This baked dinner is the ultimate comfort meal when autumn arrives. Dukkah is an Egyptian spice rub made with nuts and spices, which gives a lovely depth of texture and burst of flavour.

SERVES 4 PREP TIME: **20 MINS** COOKING TIME: **45 MINS**

2 thick slices wholegrain sourdough or gluten-free bread, torn into small pieces
3 tablespoons grated parmesan cheese
2 garlic cloves, crushed
2 tablespoons dukkah
1 tablespoon wholegrain mustard
1 tablespoon white wine vinegar
500 g (1 lb 2 oz) butternut pumpkin (squash), cut into chunks

500 g (1 lb 2 oz) desiree potatoes, cut into quarters
1 large beetroot, halved and sliced
2 teaspoons olive oil
2 tablespoons thyme leaves
600 g (1 lb 5 oz) chicken breasts
300 g (10½ oz) green beans, topped and tailed

Preheat the oven to 180°C (350°F) fan-forced. Line a baking dish and two large baking trays with baking paper.

Combine the bread, parmesan, half the garlic, the mustard, white wine vinegar and 1 tablespoon of dukkah and season well.

Spread the pumpkin, potato and beetroot on the trays in a single layer. Sprinkle with oil and thyme and season well. Roast for 25 minutes, turning occasionally, until golden and tender.

Sprinkle the bread crumble over the vegetables. Coat the chicken in the remaining garlic and dukkah and season well. Add the chicken to one of the trays and bake both trays for another 15–20 minutes until crunchy and golden and the chicken is cooked through.

Meanwhile, steam the green beans for 5 minutes or until tender.

Serve the chicken with the root vegetable crumble and green beans.

ANALYSIS SUMMARY _____

(PER SERVE) ENERGY 1949 KJ (466 CAL), PROTEIN 48 G, TOTAL FAT 11 G, SATURATED FAT 3 G, CARBOHYDRATE 38 G, SUGARS 12 G, DIETARY FIBRE 12 G

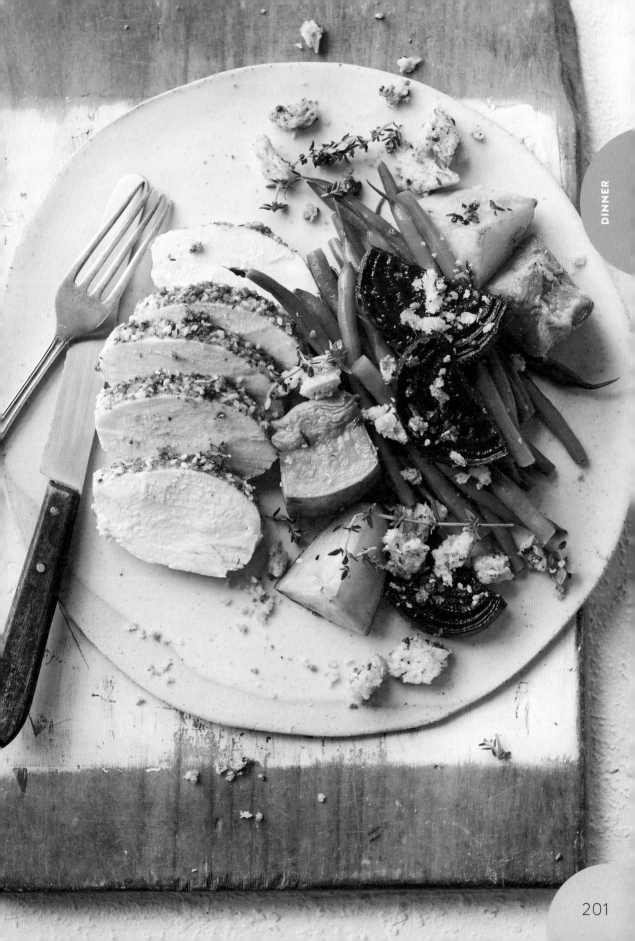

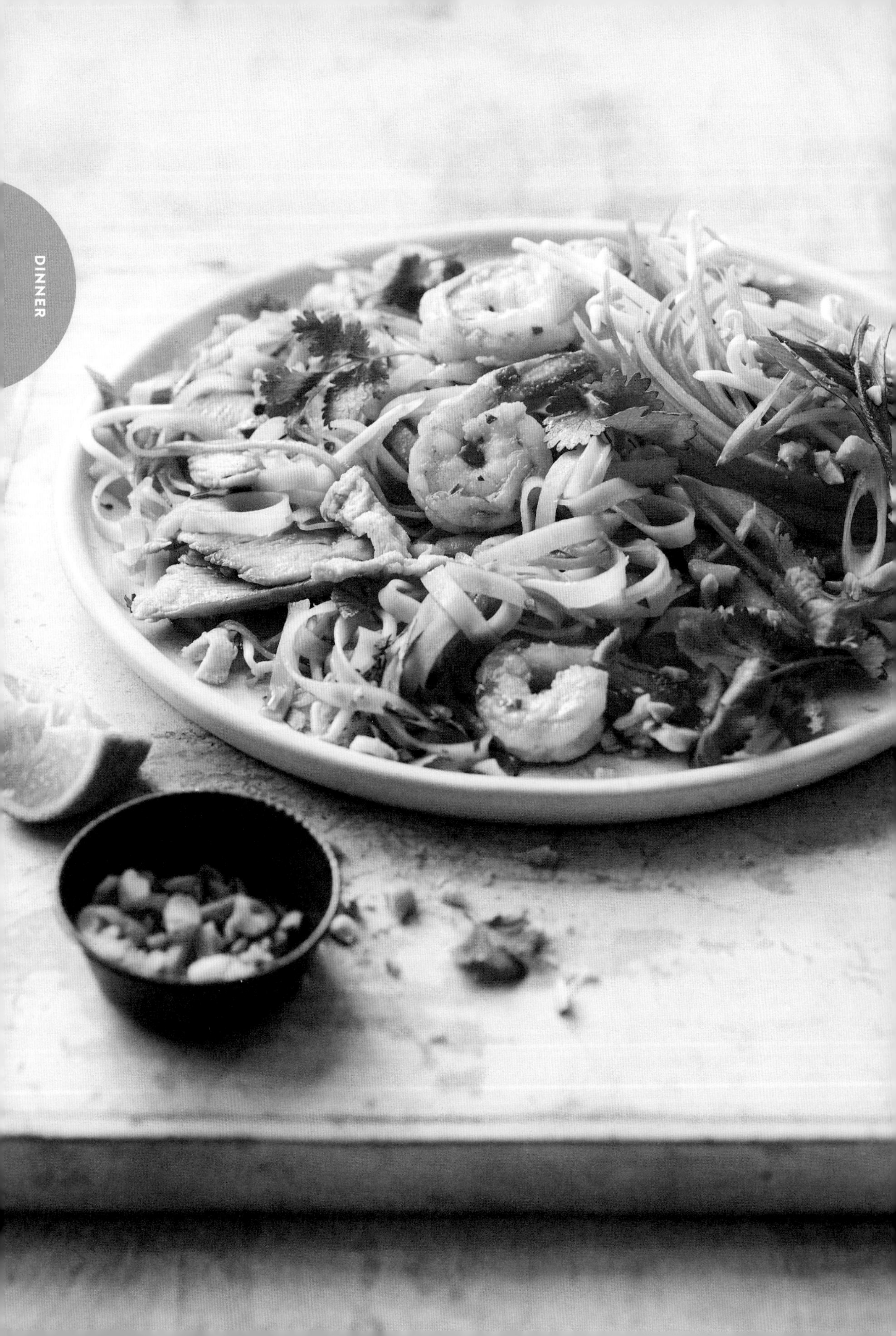

Make-at-home pad Thai

Many of us love takeaway pad Thai, but it can be very high in saturated fat and sodium. This fresh spin on a favourite packs in extra protein and veggies for a balanced meal. For a meat-free version, substitute firm tofu for the chicken and prawns. Use tamari or gluten-free soy sauce if you're gluten intolerant.

SERVES 4 PREP TIME: **20 MINS** COOKING TIME: **15 MINS**

200 g (7 oz) rice stick noodles
2 tablespoons salt-reduced soy sauce
2 tablespoons lime juice
1 tablespoon fish sauce
1 tablespoon olive oil
300 g (10 ½ oz) chicken breast, sliced
400 g (14 oz) raw prawns, peeled and deveined
2 small red chillies, seeded and finely chopped

2 carrots, shaved into ribbons
2 eggs, whisked
2 spring onions (scallions), chopped
2 cups (230 g) bean sprouts
½ bunch coriander (cilantro)
½ cup (70 g) roasted peanuts, chopped
lime wedges, to serve

Put the noodles in a glass bowl and cover with hot water. Soak until just tender, then drain.

Combine the soy sauce, lime juice and fish sauce.

Heat the oil in a wok over high heat, add the chicken and stir-fry for 5 minutes or until browned. Add the prawns and chillies and stir-fry for a further 3 minutes or until the prawns are pink.

Add the carrot, egg, rice noodles and spring onion, along with the soy sauce mixture, and stir-fry for a further 2 minutes. Throw in the bean sprouts and coriander and toss to combine.

Serve immediately with chopped peanuts and fresh lime.

ANALYSIS SUMMARY ⎯⎯⎯⎯⎯⎯⎯⎯⎯⎯⎯⎯⎯⎯⎯⎯⎯⎯⎯⎯⎯⎯
(PER SERVE) ENERGY 2210 KJ (528 CAL), PROTEIN 50 G, TOTAL FAT 15 G, SATURATED FAT 3 G, CARBOHYDRATE 44 G, SUGARS 7 G, DIETARY FIBRE 7 G

Cheeky chow mein

This healthy chow mein replaces some of the noodles with cabbage and extra vegetables, making it not only lower in carbohydrate but higher in fibre, which is great for gut health. You can also throw in any leftover vegetables that need using up. Just be careful with your sauces, however: choose salt-reduced (low-sodium) options and check for gluten if you are sensitive.

SERVES 4 PREP TIME: 5 MINS COOKING TIME: 15 MINS

2 teaspoons olive oil
1 onion, chopped
400 g (14 oz) lean beef mince
2 garlic cloves, crushed
1 tablespoon curry powder
1 cup (250 ml) salt-reduced beef stock
1 tablespoon salt-reduced soy sauce
1 tablespoon oyster sauce
150 g (5½ oz) fresh egg noodles
¼ savoy cabbage, shredded
2 carrots, chopped
200 g (7 oz) green beans, topped and tailed
1 cup (140 g) frozen peas
juice of ½ lime
lime wedges, for serving

Heat the oil in a wok or a large frying pan. Add the onion and stir-fry for 2 minutes. Add the beef mince and garlic and stir-fry for 5 minutes or until the beef starts to brown.

Add the curry powder, stock, soy sauce and oyster sauce along with the noodles, cabbage and carrot. Stir-fry for 5 minutes or until the vegetables start to soften and the noodles are tender.

Add the green beans, peas and lime juice, and cook for a further 2 minutes.

Serve immediately with lime wedges.

ANALYSIS SUMMARY

(PER SERVE) ENERGY 1798 KJ (430 CAL), PROTEIN 33 G, TOTAL FAT 13 G, SATURATED FAT 4 G, CARBOHYDRATE 40 G, SUGARS 12 G, DIETARY FIBRE 11 G

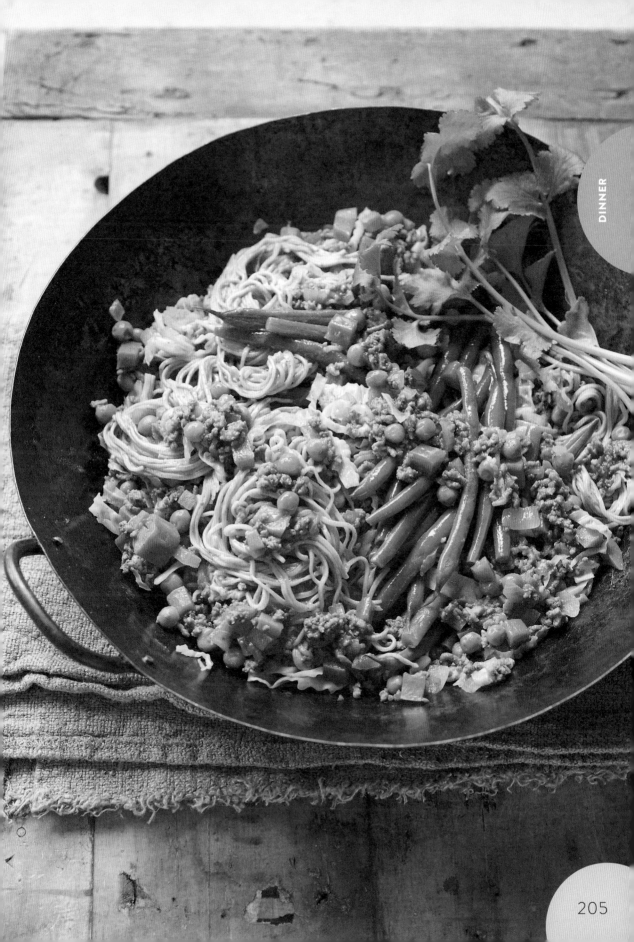

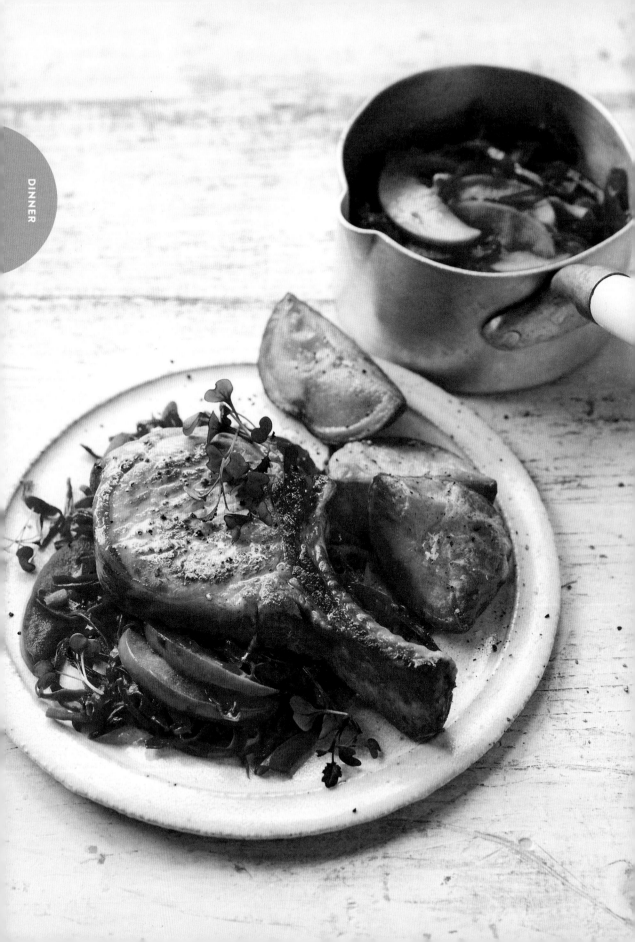

Pork chops with braised cabbage & apples : GF

Cabbage, onion and apples are great sources of the prebiotic inulin, which is important for gut health. And a healthy gut means healthy skin. But also: pork and apples ... why wouldn't you?

SERVES **4** PREP TIME: **10 MINS** COOKING TIME: **1 HR**

1 kg (2 lb 4 oz) desiree potatoes, quartered
1 tablespoon olive oil
1 cup (250 ml) apple cider
2 tablespoons red wine vinegar
1 tablespoon dijon mustard

½ red cabbage, shredded
2 onions, sliced
2 granny smith apples, cored and sliced
4 pork chops

Preheat the oven to 180°C (350°F) fan-forced and line a baking tray with baking paper.

Bring a large saucepan of water to the boil and add the potatoes. Cook for 10–15 minutes until tender, then drain. Alternatively, put the potatoes in a microwave-safe dish, cover and microwave on High for 10 minutes.

Coat the potatoes with oil, salt and pepper and arrange on the baking tray in a single layer. Bake for 40–50 minutes, turning occasionally, until crisp and golden.

Meanwhile, combine the apple cider, vinegar and mustard. Put the cabbage, onion and apples in a casserole dish and pour the cider mixture over. Cover with a lid and bake for 30 minutes. Remove the lid and bake for a further 10 minutes. Add ½ cup (125 ml) of water if it begins to dry out.

Ten minutes before the potatoes and cabbage are ready, heat a frying pan over medium heat. Season the pork chops with salt and pepper and cook for 5–10 minutes, turning, until just cooked through.

Serve the pork chops on top of the braised cabbage and apples with crispy potatoes on the side.

ANALYSIS SUMMARY

(PER SERVE) ENERGY 1805 KJ (431 CAL), PROTEIN 38 G, TOTAL FAT 10 G, SATURATED FAT 3 G, CARBOHYDRATE 41 G, SUGARS 20 G, DIETARY FIBRE 10 G

Crumbed fish with sweet potato chips & mushy peas : GF

I love these healthy fish and chips! Quinoa flakes are a crunchy gluten-free alternative to breadcrumbs – plus they provide fibre and protein. Using low-fat yoghurt is a perfect creamy replacement for mayonnaise, which can be high in saturated fat. If you are avoiding dairy, simply replace with soy or coconut yoghurt.

SERVES 4 PREP TIME: **20 MINS** COOKING TIME: **30 MINS**

500 g (1 lb 2 oz) sweet potatoes,
  cut into wedges
2 teaspoons ground cumin
1½ tablespoons olive oil
500 g (1 lb 2 oz) flathead fillets
  (or any other white fish fillets),
  cut into thick strips

1–2 eggs
½–1 cup (60–120 g) quinoa flakes
½ cup (130 g) low-fat Greek yoghurt
1 garlic clove, crushed
1 tablespoon capers, rinsed and chopped
3 tablespoons lemon juice
4 cups (560 g) frozen peas

Preheat the oven to 180°C (350°F) fan-forced and line a baking tray with baking paper. Arrange the sweet potato on the tray and sprinkle with the cumin and 2 teaspoons of oil, then season well. Cook for 25–30 minutes until golden and crisp.

Meanwhile, crumb the fish. Whisk the eggs with salt and pepper in a large bowl. Put the quinoa flakes in a separate bowl. Dip each piece of fish into the egg and then into the quinoa flakes to coat.

Heat the remaining oil in a large frying pan over medium heat. Cook the fish for 2–3 minutes on each side until crispy and golden.

Mix together the yoghurt, garlic, capers and 1 tablespoon of the lemon juice.

To make the mushy peas, cook the peas in boiling water until tender, then drain well and mash with the remaining lemon juice. Season with salt and pepper.

Serve the fish with the mushy peas and sweet potato chips, with the yoghurt tartare on the side.

ANALYSIS SUMMARY

(PER SERVE) ENERGY 2099 KJ (501 CAL), PROTEIN 44 G, TOTAL FAT 12 G, SATURATED FAT 2 G, CARBOHYDRATE 46 G, SUGARS 15 G, DIETARY FIBRE 15 G

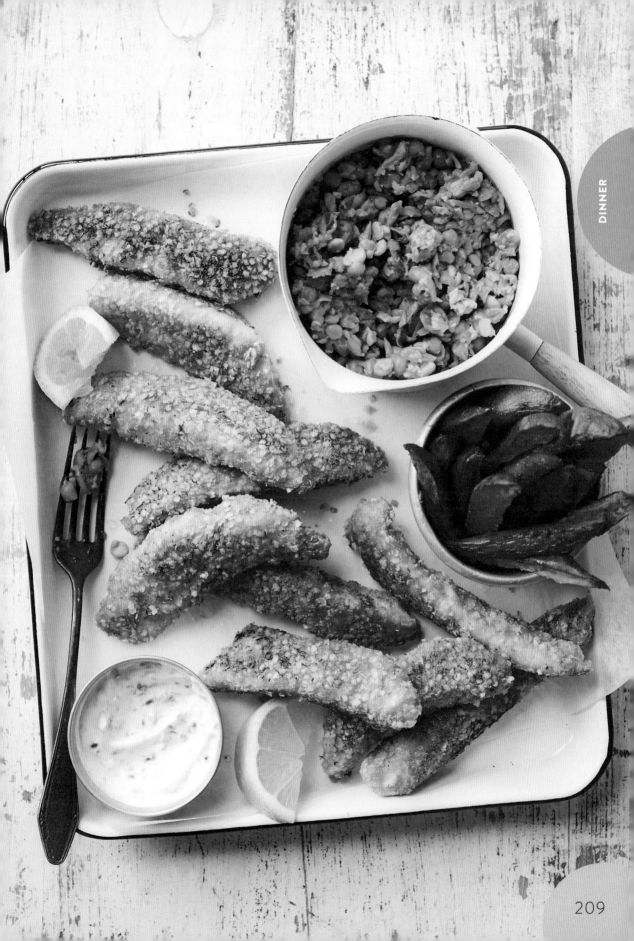

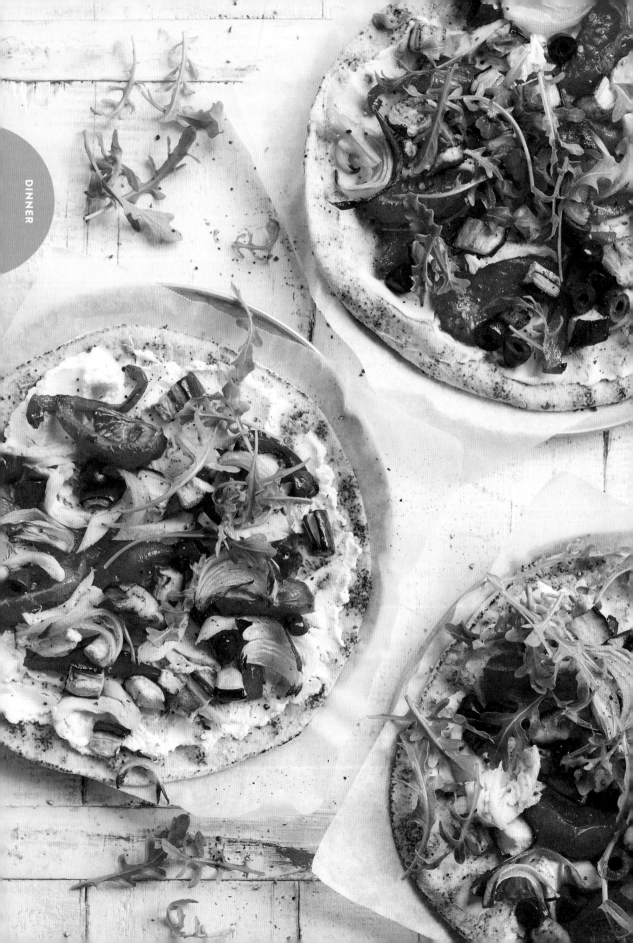

Mediterranean chicken pizza

Pizza can be a nutritious meal if you think outside the box. Leftover roast vegetables make a great topping, as does roast meat – a delicious and healthy alternative to processed meat, which is high in sodium, preservatives and saturated fat. Unless you are avoiding dairy, there is no reason to avoid cheese! Choosing reduced-fat feta, cheddar and ricotta is a smarter way to bump up the protein in your meals.

SERVES 4 PREP TIME: **20 MINS** COOKING TIME: **40 MINS**

1 eggplant (aubergine), cut into cubes
1 onion, cut into wedges
1 red capsicum (pepper), seeded and cut into wedges
3 tomatoes, cut into wedges
½ cup (90 g) black olives
400 g (14 oz) chicken breasts
2 teaspoons olive oil
4 large wholemeal pitta breads or gluten-free wraps
1 cup (230 g) reduced-fat ricotta cheese
1 cup (35 g) rocket (arugula)

Preheat the oven to 180°C (350°F) fan-forced and line two baking trays with baking paper. Put the eggplant, onion, capsicum and tomato on one tray and season with salt and pepper. Bake for 20–30 minutes until browned.

Meanwhile, put the chicken breasts on the other tray. Drizzle with the oil and season with salt and pepper. Bake for 15–20 minutes, then shred the chicken.

When you're almost ready to eat, lay the bread in a single layer on two baking trays. Spread 3 tablespoons of ricotta over each pitta bread and top with roasted vegetables, olives and shredded chicken. Bake for 10 minutes or until the bread is crispy.

Serve with rocket scattered on top.

ANALYSIS SUMMARY

(PER SERVE) ENERGY 1897 KJ (434 CAL), PROTEIN 42 G, TOTAL FAT 11 G, SATURATED FAT 3 G, CARBOHYDRATE 41 G, SUGARS 12 G, DIETARY FIBRE 10 G

Pasta with chicken, roasted peppers & goat's cheese

Pasta often gets the blame for expanding waistlines, but context is key when it comes to carbs. Wholemeal pasta retains more fibre, B vitamins and minerals vital for healthy skin. When combined with adequate protein and vegetables, pasta can make for a low-GI, balanced and healthy meal. There are also some great high-fibre and gluten-free pastas available.

SERVES **4** PREP TIME: **20 MINS** COOKING TIME: **40 MINS**

200 g (7 oz) wholemeal penne pasta
400 g (14 oz) jar roasted red capsicum (pepper)
2 garlic cloves, crushed
1 tablespoon red wine vinegar
1 large handful basil, chopped
1 tablespoon olive oil
400 g (14 oz) chicken breasts, cut into strips
150 g (5½ oz) baby spinach
100 g (3½ oz) goat's cheese, cubed

Cook the pasta in a large saucepan of boiling water, following the packet directions, until al dente. Drain.

Put the roasted capsicum, garlic, vinegar and half the basil in a blender and blend until smooth.

Heat the oil in a non-stick frying pan over medium heat and sauté the chicken strips, in batches, for 5 minutes or until golden. Remove from the pan and set aside.

Pour the capsicum sauce into the same pan and add the pasta and baby spinach. Warm through for 5 minutes, then stir in the chicken, remaining basil and the goat's cheese.

Spoon into bowls and enjoy straightaway.

ANALYSIS SUMMARY _____

(PER SERVE) ENERGY 2046 KJ (489 CAL), PROTEIN 42 G, TOTAL FAT 12 G, SATURATED FAT 5 G, CARBOHYDRATE 49 G, SUGARS 16 G, DIETARY FIBRE 9 G

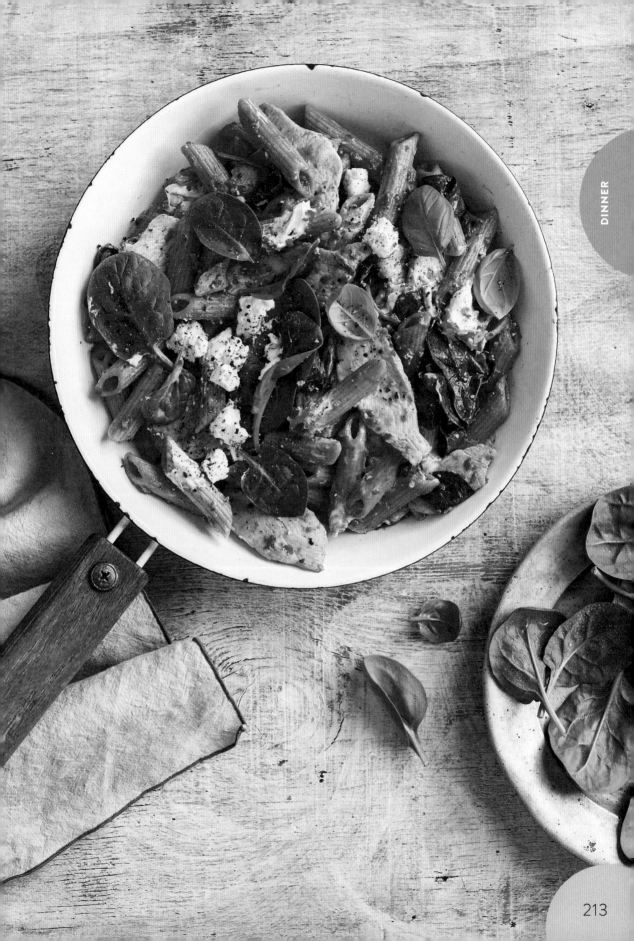

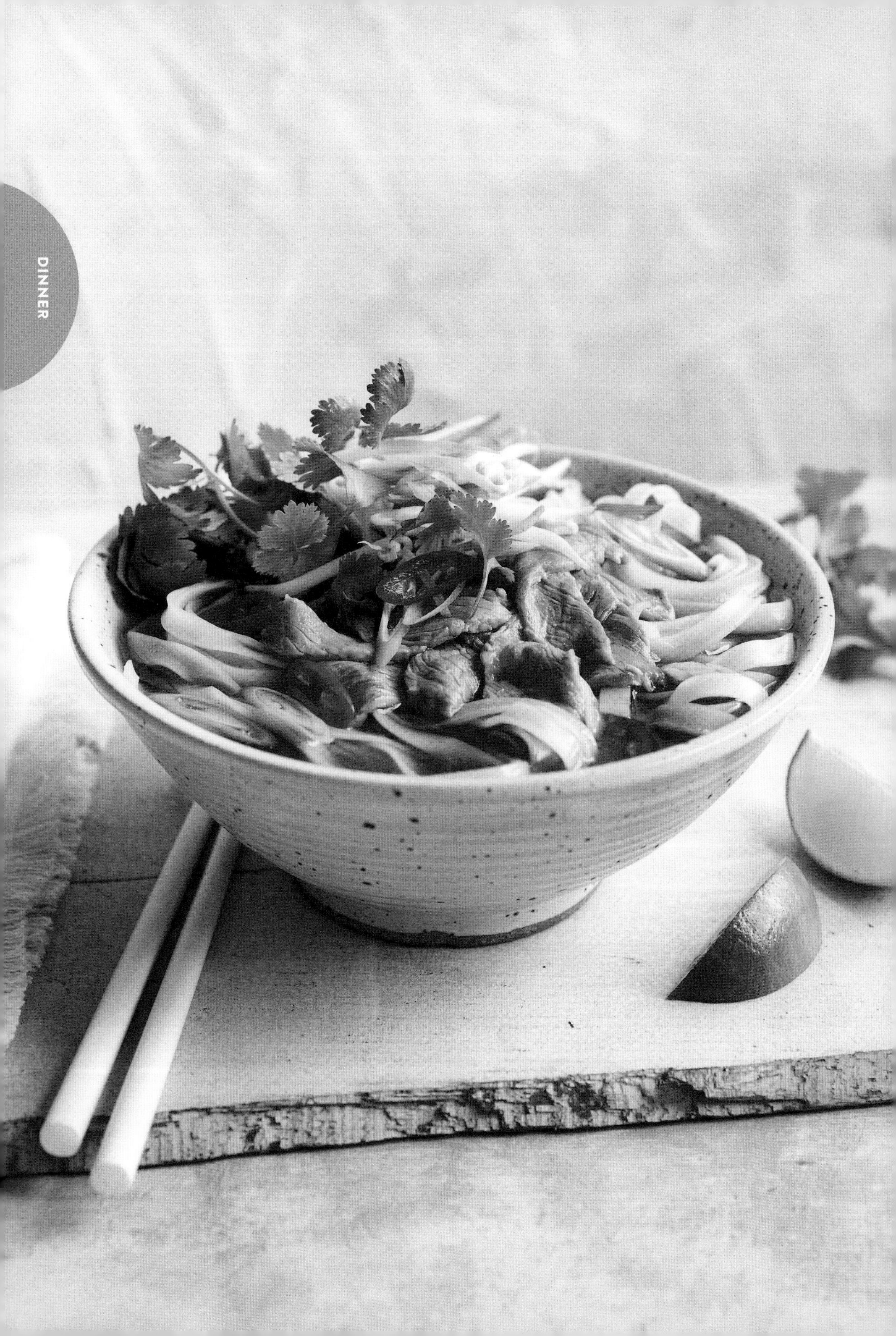

Fool's pho : GF

This is a cheat's version for a super-quick, comforting and nourishing meal that is gluten free, low-GI and high in lean protein. The broth is an important component here, so go for a good-quality stock or bone broth, and make sure your soy sauce is gluten free. This recipe uses Japanese soba noodles made from buckwheat, a nutritious gluten-free seed, making it much higher in fibre and lower GI than traditional rice noodles.

SERVES 2 PREP TIME: **5 MINS** COOKING TIME: **10 MINS**

250 g (9 oz) lean sirloin steak
100 g (3½ oz) rice stick noodles
1 cup (115 g) bean sprouts
1 large handful Thai basil or coriander
    (cilantro), chopped
1 spring onion (scallion), chopped
1 red chilli, seeded and finely chopped
1 lime, cut into wedges

BROTH
2 star anise
1 cinnamon stick
½ teaspoon coriander seeds
2 cups (500 ml) good-quality salt-reduced
    beef stock or bone broth
2 teaspoons gluten-free soy sauce
2 teaspoons fish sauce
1 teaspoon sesame oil
1 small knob of ginger

Put the beef in the freezer for 15 minutes, while you prepare the other components. This will make it easier to slice thinly.

For the broth, put the star anise, cinnamon and coriander seeds in a saucepan over medium heat and dry toast for 1 minute until fragrant. Pour in the stock or broth and add the soy sauce, fish sauce, sesame oil and ginger. Simmer for 10 minutes.

While the broth is simmering, put the rice noodles in a bowl and cover with boiling water. Leave them to soak for 7 minutes so they start to separate. Drain, then rinse in cold water.

Meanwhile, remove the beef from the freezer and slice into thin strips.

To serve, divide the noodles between two bowls and top with the raw beef slices in a single layer. Ladle the hot stock into each bowl over the beef to cook it, then garnish with the bean sprouts, herbs, spring onion, chilli and lime wedges.

ANALYSIS SUMMARY _____

(PER SERVE) ENERGY 1625 KJ (388 CAL), PROTEIN 39 G, TOTAL FAT 8 G, SATURATED FAT 2 G, CARBOHYDRATE 38 G, SUGARS 5 G, DIETARY FIBRE 4 G

White bean soup with kale pesto : GF

White beans are the star of this dish. They're high in resistant starch for healthy digestion, as well as B-group vitamins, plus they're gluten free. The peppery, zesty pesto gives this soup its vibrancy – and an added punch of antioxidants.

SERVES **4** PREP TIME: **10 MINS** COOKING TIME: **25 MINS**

1 teaspoon olive oil
2 onions, chopped
1 garlic clove, crushed
2 zucchini (courgettes), diced
2 x 400 g (14 oz) tins cannellini beans,
    drained and rinsed
2 litres salt-reduced vegetable stock
½ cup (130 g) low-fat Greek yoghurt

KALE PESTO
½ bunch kale, stalks removed
    and leaves chopped
1 handful basil leaves
30 g (1 oz) parmesan
30 g (1 oz) slivered almonds
1 tablespoon extra virgin olive oil
juice of 1 lemon
½ garlic clove, crushed

Heat the olive oil in a large saucepan over medium heat and sauté the onion for 3–5 minutes until starting to soften. Add the garlic and zucchini and cook for another 3 minutes, stirring often. Add the drained beans and stock, and simmer for 15 minutes. Remove from the heat and allow to cool slightly, then transfer to a food processor and blend until smooth.

Meanwhile, prepare the kale pesto. Put all the ingredients, except a few basil leaves, in a small food processer and blend until a paste begins to form. If the paste is too thick, add a tablespoon or two of water to loosen it.

Divide the soup among four bowls, then dollop a spoonful of yoghurt and a drizzle of pesto on top and swirl through. Serve immediately with the extra basil leaves on top.

ANALYSIS SUMMARY

(PER SERVE) ENERGY 1617 KJ (387 CAL), PROTEIN 22 G, TOTAL FAT 13 G, SATURATED FAT 3 G, CARBOHYDRATE 33 G, SUGARS 9 G, DIETARY FIBRE 17 G

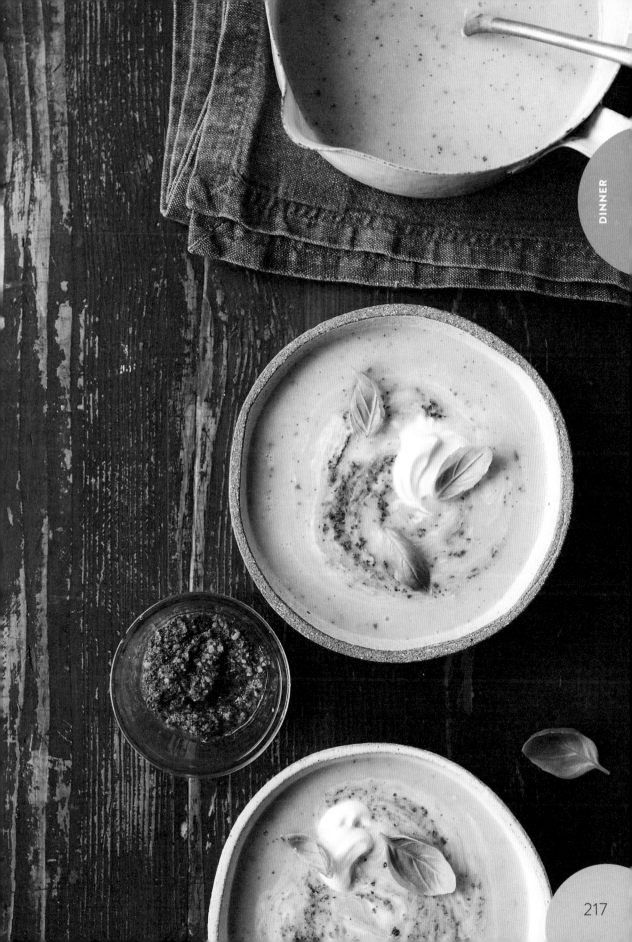

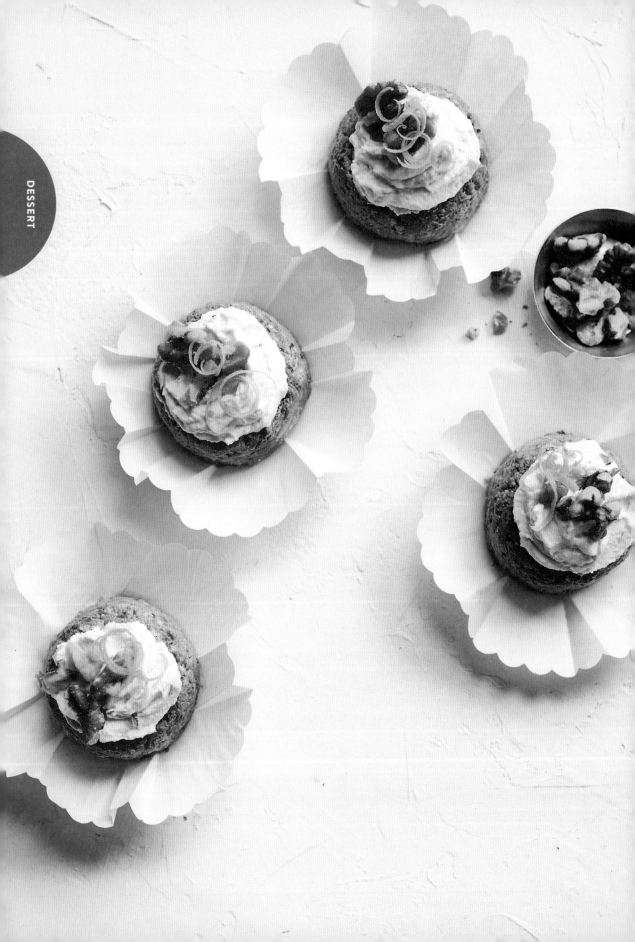

Raw carrot cake with lemon ricotta frosting : GF

This gluten-free cake is high in good fats, including monounsaturated fats and omega-3. Note that while these are great for healthy skin and heart, all fats should be eaten in moderation as part of a balanced diet.

SERVES **4** PREP TIME: **10 MINS** REFRIGERATION TIME: **20 MINS**

½ cup (85 g) pitted medjool dates, chopped
2 tablespoons chia seeds
1 cup (115 g) walnut halves
3 tablespoons shredded coconut
½ teaspoon ground cinnamon
½ teaspoon nutmeg
2 cups (310 g) grated carrot

FROSTING
200 g (7 oz) reduced-fat ricotta cheese
juice and grated zest of ½ lemon
1 tablespoon maple syrup

Mix together the dates, chia seeds and 3 tablespoons of warm water in a small bowl. Soak for at least 5 minutes.

Set aside a small handful of walnuts for decorating, then blitz the remaining walnuts in a food processor for 30 seconds. Add the soaked dates, chia seeds and water to the bowl and process again until a paste forms. Add the coconut, cinnamon and nutmeg and process again for 30 seconds.

Transfer the walnut and date mixture to a large bowl and add the grated carrot. Mix well.

Spoon the mixture into a lined shallow baking tin or individual ramekins and refrigerate while you make the frosting.

To make the frosting, use the same food processor to blend the ricotta, lemon juice and zest and maple syrup until smooth.

Using a spatula, spread the ricotta icing on top of the cake and refrigerate for at least 20 minutes to set. Decorate with the reserved chopped walnuts before serving.

ANALYSIS SUMMARY _____

(**PER SERVE**) ENERGY 1824 KJ (436 CAL), PROTEIN 11 G, TOTAL FAT 32 G, SATURATED FAT 6 G, CARBOHYDRATE 23 G, SUGARS 22 G, DIETARY FIBRE 10 G

Choc banana soft-serve : GF

This dairy-free treat hits the sweet spot if you're craving ice cream. It's a really good idea to keep peeled bananas on hand in the freezer for such moments! With a light, fluffy and creamy soft-serve texture, it's also high in potassium from the bananas, while the cacao powder provides a rich source of antioxidants and can help with cell regeneration.

SERVES **4** PREP TIME: **5 MINS**

2 bananas, chopped and frozen
2 tablespoons cacao powder
1 tablespoon maple syrup
½ cup (50 g) vanilla protein powder
30 g (1 oz) cacao nibs
30 g (1 oz) flaked almonds

Put the banana, cacao powder, maple syrup and protein powder in a small food processor and blend until smooth and creamy.

Spoon into glasses or cups, top with cacao nibs and flaked almonds and serve immediately.

ANALYSIS SUMMARY ———————————————————————
(PER SERVE) ENERGY 783 KJ (187 CAL), PROTEIN 9 G, TOTAL FAT 8 G, SATURATED FAT 3 G, CARBOHYDRATE 19 G, SUGARS 13 G, DIETARY FIBRE 3 G

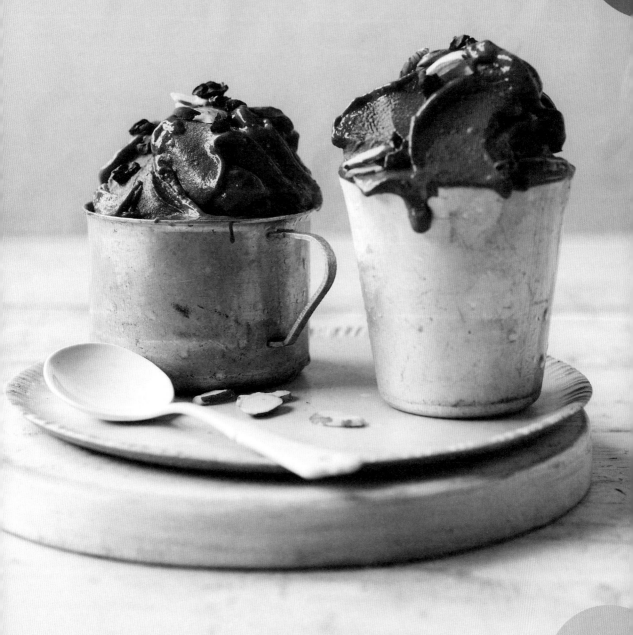

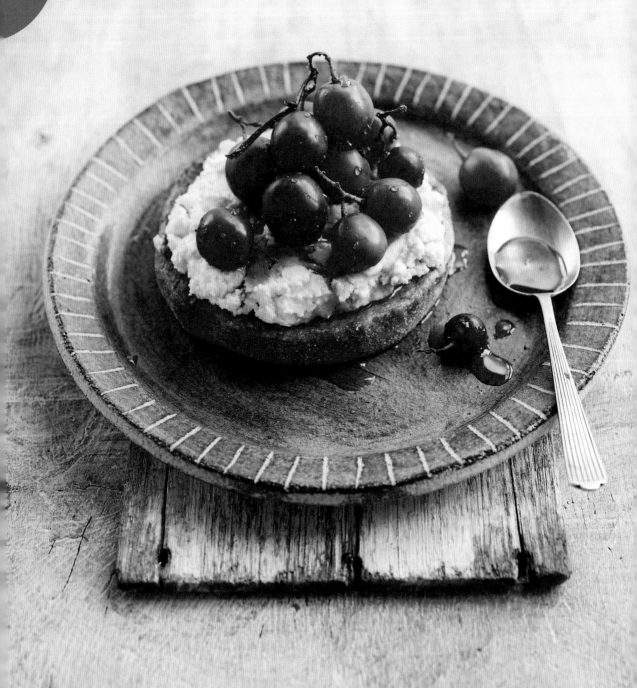

Roasted grapes with ricotta & French toast

Traditionally, French toast is high in added sugars and saturated fat, but by making a few smart changes it can be a delicious source of low-GI carbohydrate, protein and calcium. So you can have your dessert and tick off those important food groups too! Pomegranate molasses is a staple in Middle Eastern cooking. The sweet and sour syrup is made by reducing pomegranate juice. It's a great alternative to added sugar, but if you can't find it, use maple syrup instead.

SERVES **2** PREP TIME: **5 MINS** COOKING TIME: **20 MINS**

200 g (7 oz) red grapes
1 large egg
100 ml (3½ fl oz) skim milk
1 teaspoon ground cinnamon
olive oil spray
1 wholegrain or gluten-free English muffin,
 cut in half through the middle
200 g (7 oz) reduced-fat ricotta cheese
1 tablespoon pomegranate molasses (or maple syrup)

Preheat the oven to 180°C (350°F) fan-forced and line a baking tray with baking paper. Spread the grapes on the tray and roast for 15–20 minutes until softened.

Meanwhile, whisk together the egg, milk and cinnamon in a bowl.

Heat a non-stick frying pan over medium heat and spray lightly with olive oil spray.

Dip the muffin halves into the egg mixture, evenly coating both sides and shaking off any excess. Cook for 2–3 minutes on each side until lightly browned.

Serve each muffin half topped with ricotta and grapes. Drizzle with pomegranate molasses or maple syrup.

ANALYSIS SUMMARY

(PER SERVE) ENERGY 1229 KJ (294 CAL), PROTEIN 17 G, TOTAL FAT 6 G, SATURATED FAT 3 G, CARBOHYDRATE 39 G, SUGARS 26 G, DIETARY FIBRE 4 G

Fig & brazil nut bombs : GF

Brazil nuts are very high in selenium, an anti-inflammatory antioxidant that supports cell regeneration and healthy thyroid function. You could substitute almonds, walnuts, pumpkin seeds or sunflower seeds here, which are also packed full of poly- and monounsaturated fats that nourish and hydrate the skin from the inside out.

MAKES **8 SMALL BALLS** PREP TIME: **20 MINS** REFRIGERATION TIME: **30 MINS**

½ cup (95 g) dried figs, stems trimmed, chopped
½ cup (75 g) brazil nuts
3 tablespoons vanilla or chocolate protein powder,
   plus extra if necessary
2 tablespoons cacao powder
2 teaspoons ground ginger
pinch of salt
2 tablespoons cacao nibs

Put the figs in a bowl, cover with hot water and leave to soak for 5–10 minutes.

Meanwhile, pulse the brazil nuts in a food processor to make a coarse meal. Add the protein powder, cacao powder, ginger and salt.

Drain the figs, keeping the liquid, then add the figs to the food processor. Process into a uniform, crumbly 'dough'. If it is too dry, add the reserved liquid, a little at a time, and process until the dough comes together. If too wet, add more protein powder.

Form tablespoons of dough into balls with your hands, then roll in the cacao nibs to coat.

Refrigerate for at least 30 minutes before eating.

ANALYSIS SUMMARY ————————————————

(PER SERVE) ENERGY 1221 KJ (292 CAL), PROTEIN 8 G, TOTAL FAT 19 G, SATURATED FAT 6 G, CARBOHYDRATE 20 G, SUGARS 17 G, DIETARY FIBRE 7 G

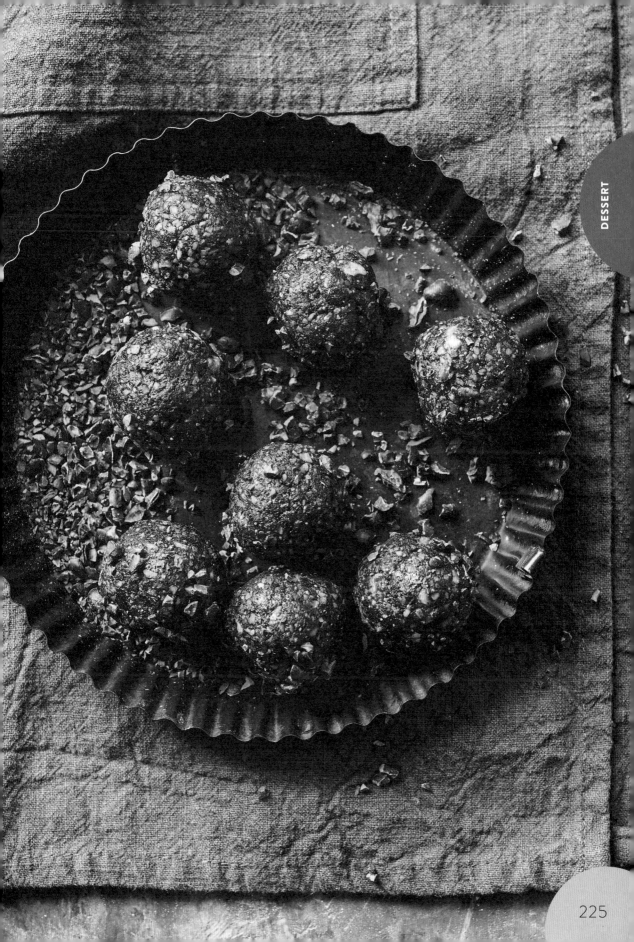

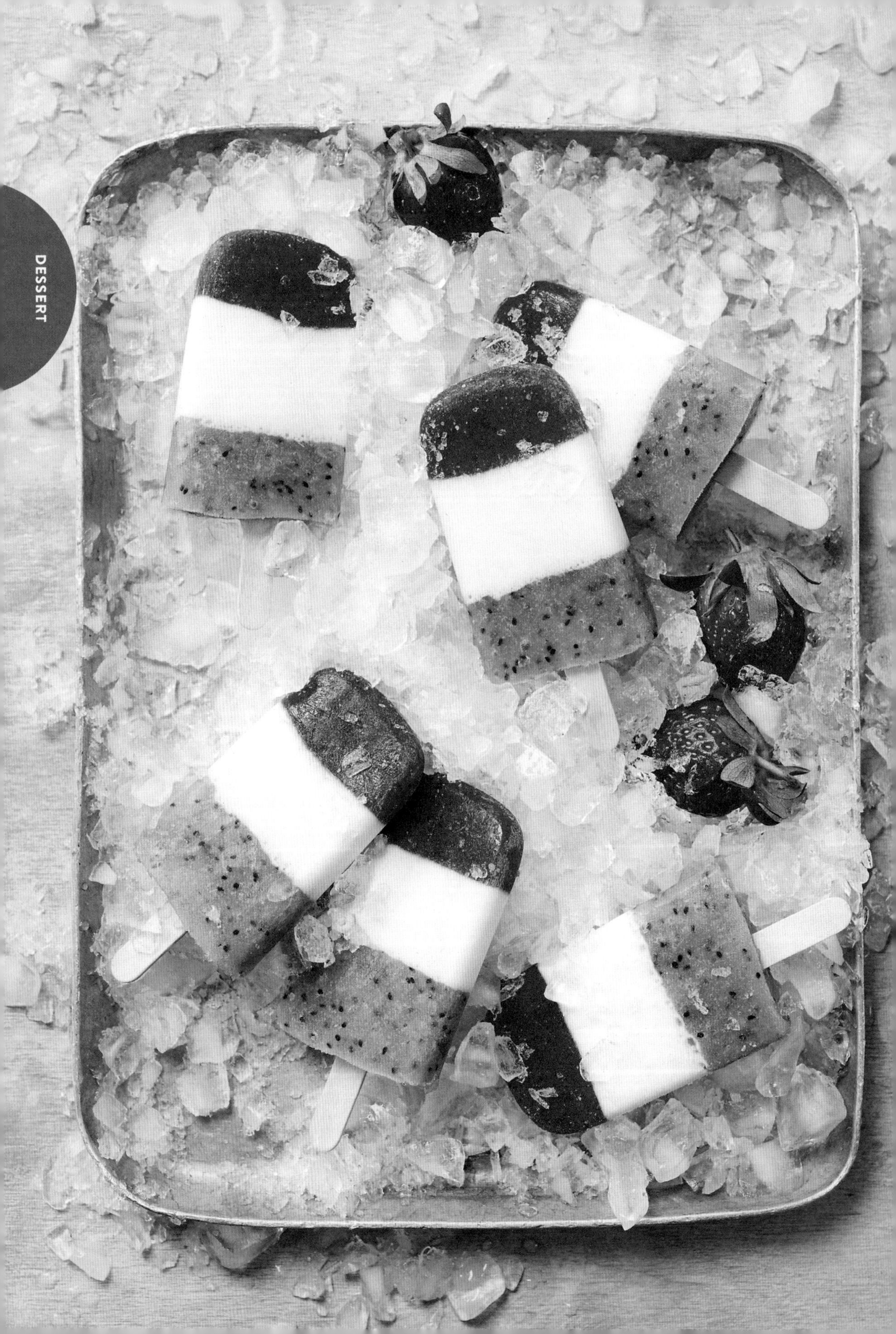

Kiwifruit, strawberry & basil pops : GF

These icy pops are perfect as a refreshing palate cleanser after a main meal or a snack. To boost the protein content, just add vanilla protein powder to the yoghurt. Because there is no added sugar, they may freeze harder than commercial popsicles, so just leave them to thaw for a little longer.

MAKES AROUND **6 POPS**   PREP TIME: **20 MINS**   FREEZING TIME: **5–10 HOURS**

1 cup (150 g) fresh or frozen strawberries
grated zest and juice of 1 lime
1 cup (260 g) low-fat Greek yoghurt
1 tablespoon honey
4 kiwifruit, peeled and diced
1 small handful basil leaves

Put the strawberries and half the lime zest and juice in a food processor and blitz until smooth. Spoon into 6 popsicle moulds, insert sticks and freeze for several hours until set.

Mix the yoghurt and honey until well combined. Spoon into the moulds and freeze for several hours.

Put the kiwifruit, remaining lime zest and juice and the basil leaves in the food processor and blitz until smooth. Spoon into the moulds and freeze for at least 5 hours or overnight until completely set.

To remove the pops, put the moulds in room-temperature water for a few minutes until the ices can be wriggled free.

ANALYSIS SUMMARY _____

(PER SERVE) ENERGY 634 KJ (152 CAL), PROTEIN 7 G, TOTAL FAT 2 G, SATURATED FAT 1 G, CARBOHYDRATE 23 G, SUGARS 23 G, DIETARY FIBRE 5 G

Index

Recipe index

FURTHER READING AND REFERENCES

I consulted hundreds of scientific studies, articles and websites during the research for this book. For a complete list of references, please visit the Murdoch Books website (murdochbooks.com.au) and search for Healthy Skin Diet.

Published in 2020 by Murdoch Books, an imprint of Allen & Unwin

Murdoch Books Australia
83 Alexander Street,
Crows Nest NSW 2065
Phone: +61 (0)2 8425 0100
murdochbooks.com.au
info@murdochbooks.com.au

Murdoch Books UK
Ormond House, 26–27 Boswell Street,
London, WC1N 3JZ
Phone: +44 (0) 20 8785 5995
murdochbooks.co.uk
info@murdochbooks.co.uk

For corporate orders & custom publishing contact our business development team at salesenquiries@murdochbooks.com.au

Publisher: Jane Morrow
Editorial Manager: Jane Price
Creative Manager: Vivien Valk
Designers: Trisha Garner, Susanne Geppert
Editors: Melody Lord, Ariane Durkin
Photographer: Chris Chen, apart from pages 4–5, 13, 33, 37, 64 (Shutterstock), 11, 50 (iStock) and 16, 31, 46 (Adobe Stock)
Stylist: Vanessa Austin
Food preparation at shoot: Tracy Rutherford
Illustrations for case studies: Cécile Parker
Production Director: Lou Playfair

Text © Geraldine Georgeou 2020
Design © Murdoch Books 2020
Photography © Chris Chen, unless specified

ISBN 978 1 76052 490 6 Australia
ISBN 978 1 76052 570 5 UK

A catalogue record for this book is available from the National Library of Australia

A catalogue record for this book is available from the British Library

Colour reproduction by Splitting Image Colour Studio Pty Ltd, Clayton, Victoria
Printed by C & C Offset Printing Co Ltd, China

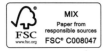